Questions and Answers Set:

Book 2
2018 Edition

By Stu Silverstein, M.D., FAAP

MedHumor Medical Publications, LLC.

www.passtheboards.com

MedHumor Medical Publications, Stamford, Connecticut

Medhumor
Medical Publications, LLC.
www.passtheboards.com

Published by:
Medhumor Medical Publications, LLC
1127 High Ridge Road, Suite 332
Stamford, CT 06905 U.S.A.

All rights reserved. No part of this book may be reproduced, or transmitted in any form or by any means, electronic or mechanical, including photocopying, recording or by any information storage and retrieval system without written permission from the author, except for the inclusion of brief quotations in a review.
One-panel cartoons are copyright ©·2000 Medhumor Medical Publications, LLC.

Copyright © 2002, 2008, 2016, 2018 Medhumor Medical Publications, LLC

ISBN: **978-1-7320780-9-3**

First Edition Copyright © 2002 Medhumor Medical Publications, LLC
Second Edition Copyright © 2008 Medhumor Medical Publications, LLC
Third Edition Copyright © 2016 Medhumor Medical Publications, LLC
2018 Edition Copyright © 2018 Medhumor Medical Publications, LLC

Printed in the United States of America

This book is designed to provide information and guidance in regard to the subject matter covered. It is to be used as a study guide for physicians preparing for the General Pediatric Certifying Exam administered by the American Board of Pediatrics. It is not meant to be a clinical manual. The reader is advised to consult textbooks and other reference manuals in making clinical decisions. It is not the purpose of this book to reprint all the information that is otherwise available, but rather to assist the Board Candidate in organizing the material to facilitate study and recall on the exam. The reader is encouraged to read other sources of material, in particular picture atlases that are available.

Although every precaution has been taken in the preparation of this book, the publisher, author, and members of the editorial board assume no responsibility for errors, omissions or typographical mistakes. Neither is any liability assumed for damages resulting from the direct and indirect use of the information contained herein. The book contains information that is up-to-date only up to the printing date. Due to the very nature of the medical profession, there will be points out-of-date as soon as the book rolls off the press. The purpose of this book is to educate and entertain.

**If you do not wish to be bound by the above,
you may return this book to the publisher for a full refund.**

Publisher:	MedHumor Medical Publications, LLC Stamford, CT
VP/Content Development :	Stuart Silverstein, MD, FAAP Clinical Director Firefly After Hours Pediatrics, LLC Stamford, CT Assistant Clinical Professor Emergency Medicine New York Medical College
Senior Editor:	Lourdes Geise, MD, FAAP
Vice President/ Operations:	Brian Cahn 3rd Year Medical Student Albert Einstein College of Medicine
Design / Copy Editor:	Antoinette D'Amore, A.D. Design addesign@videotron.ca
Cover Designer:	Rachel Mindrup www.rmindrup.com Leo Rosas Vickers www.leorosasvickers.com

About the Author

Dr. Stu Silverstein is the founder and CEO of Medhumor Medical Publications, LLC which began with the publication of the critically acclaimed "Laughing your way to Passing the Pediatric Boards"™ back in the spring of 2000. Word spread quickly that finally there was a book out there that turned a traditionally daunting process into one that was actually fun and enjoyable. This groundbreaking study guide truly "Took the Boredom out of Board review"® with reports from our readers that they were able to reduce their study and review time in half. Those who were taking the exam for the 2nd time not only passed but increased their scores dramatically.

Their supplementary pediatric titles have also been crtically acclaimed. Medhumor Publications LLC, has since expanded their catalogue to include a title for the USMLE Step 3, Neonatology and the Neurolgy Board exams.

The concept of the "Laughing your way to Passing the Boards"™ and Medhumor Medical Publications, LLC were conceived by Dr. Silverstein. He brought his years of experience in the field of Standup Comedy and Comedy writing after he realized the critical need for a study guide that spoke the language of colleagues rather than the language of dusty textbooks. His work as a Standup Comedian and Medical Humorist has frequently been featured in several newspapers, radio programs and TV shows, including the New York Times, WCBS newsradio in NY City, as well as World News Tonight with Peter Jennings.

Dr. Silverstein has also served as a contributing editor for the Resident and Staff Physician annual board review issue and has authored numerous articles on medical humor. He has served on the faculty of the Osler Institute Board Review course, UCLA Pediatric Board Review course and several local board review courses. He is the co-author of "What about Me? Growing up with a Developmentally Disabled Sibling" written with Dr. Bryna Siegel, professor of Child Psychiatry , the University of California San Francisco. Dr. Silverstein is in demand as a lecturer for residency programs on successful preparation for the pediatric board exam.

In addition to writing, lecturing, and expanding the scope of Medhumor Medical Publications, LLC., Dr. Silverstein is the Medical Director for Firefly After Hours Pediatrics, a subacute emergency practice. Dr. Silverstein is an Assistant Clinical Professor of Emergency Medicine at the New York Medical College in Valhalla, New York.

Questions and Answers Volume 2 (3rd Edition)

In putting together the 3rd edition of our *Question and Answer* series we did our utmost to incorporate the suggestions of our readers who successfully passed the General Pediatric Board Exam as well as the Recertification Exam.

Each book now contains 400 questions each broken down by subspecialty. This allows the reader to focus on areas that need improvement.

All questions have been reviewed and revised based on the content specifications published by the American Academy of Pediatrics and the American Board of Pediatrics. All outdated questions and answers have been replaced with new questions. The subspecialty list matches the subspecialty list in our Main Pediatric Study Guide. We have added a section on Ethics for the Primary care Pediatrician as well as Patient Safety and Quality Improvement.

We hope that this updated *Question and Answer* book will continue to serve those for whom passing the Pediatric Certification or getting through the Pediatric MOC process is the next ticket to be punched.

—Stuart Silverstein, MD, FAAP
Stamford, CT

Table of Contents

Questions 1

- Growth and Development 3
- Nutrition 5
- Preventive Pediatrics 9
- Poisons and Toxins 11
- Fetus and Newborn 13
- Fluids and Lytes 20
- Genetics 24
- Allergy and Immunology 28
- Infectious Disease 31
- Inborn Errors of Metabolism 40
- Endocrinology 43
- GI 49
- Pulmonary 54
- Cardiology 59
- Heme onc 66
- Renal 73
- Urinary 77
- Neurology 79
- Musculoskeletal 84
- Dermatology 89
- Rheumatology 92
- Ophthalmology 95

Questions and Answers

ENT 97
Adolescent Medicine and Gynecology 101
Sports Medicine 104
Substance Abuse 105
Disorders of Cognition, Language and Learning 107
Behavior and Mental Health 110
Psychosocial 111
Critical Care 118
Emergency Medicine 120
Pharmacology and Pain management 127
Research and Statistics 128
Ethics for Primary Care Physicians 132
Patient Safety and Quality Improvement 134

Answers 137

Growth and Development 139
Nutrition 141
Preventive Pediatrics 145
Poisons and Toxins 146
Fetus and Newborn 147
Fluids and Lytes 153
Genetics 156
Allergy and Immunology 159
Infectious Disease 161
Inborn Errors of Metabolism 168

Section	Page
Endocrinology	170
GI	175
Pulmonary	179
Cardiology	182
Heme onc	187
Renal	193
Urinary	196
Neurology	198
Musculoskeletal	202
Dermatology	206
Rheumatology	208
Ophthalmology	211
ENT	213
Adolescent Medicine and Gynecology	216
Sports Medicine	218
Substance Abuse	219
Disorders of Cognition, Language and Learning	221
Behavior and Mental Health	223
Psychosocial	225
Critical Care	231
Emergency Medicine	233
Pharmacology and Pain management	238
Research and Statistics	239
Ethics for Primary Care Physicians	242
Patient Safety and Quality Improvement	244

Questions

Growth and Development

1) At the 18 month routine well child examination you note that the head circumference has remained at the 45th percentile for age and the height has remained at the 50th percentile for age for the last 6 months. Mom is concerned because her son doesn't eat enough and has become increasingly pickier. He is now below the 5th percentile for weight. He was at the 35th percentile for weight at the 12 month visit when whole milk was introduced. There are no chronic illnesses, and he has been very healthy other than the occasional cough and cold. All immunizations are current. Physical exam is otherwise normal. Each of the following interventions would be appropriate in this setting *except*:

    A) Admission for observation of his feeding and growing
    B) Occupational therapy consultation
    C) Social services consultation
    D) Behavioral health specialty consultation
    E) Nutritional consultation

2) Which of the following is true regarding monitoring of growth during the first 2 years of life?

    A) World Health Organization (WHO) growth charts correlate with optimal growth in formula fed infants
    B) US Center for Disease Control (CDC) growth charts correlate with optimal growth in breast fed infants
    C) World Health Organization (WHO) growth charts should be used to assess growth of children younger than 2 years of age
    D) US Center for Disease Control (CDC) growth charts should be used to assess growth of children younger than 2 years of age
    E) Height at 2 months of age correlates well with mean parental height.

3) Each of the following statements is true regarding growth failure in children with chronic kidney disease except :

A) Improved nutrition and supplementation can result in improved linear growth rates
B) Metabolic bone disease can impair linear growth
C) Prolonged steroid use decreases growth hormone secretion and liver production of IGF-1
D) Dialysis improves growth but does not result in catch up growth
E) Renal transplantation improves growth and allows for catch up growth

4) Which of the following would be appropriate as a screen for a general mental health condition in a 13 year old during a routine well visit in a general pediatric office setting?

A) The Patient Health Questionnaire (PHQ-9)
B) The Child Behavior Checklist (CBCL)
C) The LMAO Scale (Lexington Mental Agility Online)
D) Ages and Stages Questionnaire® (ASQ)
E) The Pediatric Symptom Checklist (PSC)

5) Which of the following is sufficient in determining that a two year old child is at high risk for obesity?

A) Weight greater than the 90th percentile for age
B) Height greater than the 90th percentile for age
C) BMI greater than the 85th percentile for age
D) Weight greater than the 85th percentile for age and family history of diabetes
E) Large for gestational age at birth

Nutrition

6) Which of the following statements regarding breast-feeding is *TRUE*?

A) Breast-feeding through the first 6 months of life is adequate
B) The components of breast milk remain constant through the first year
C) Breast milk provides protection against infection primarily through IgG and passive immunity
D) Human milk contains activated T cells and alpha interferon
E) Human milk likely complements the infant's own immune system via immunomodulation

7) During the first 6 months of life, which of the following can be obtained exclusively with breast milk under *ALL* conditions?

A) Phylloquinone
B) Fluoride
C) Vitamin D
D) Ascorbic Acid
E) Vitamin B12

8) Match the numbered descriptions on the left with the forms of Vitamin D on the right.

1) Ergocalciferol
2) Cholecalciferol
3) Hydroxylated in the liver
4) Activated calcitriol
5) Hydroxylated in the kidney

(A) 1,25 hydroxy vitamin D
(B) 25, hydroxy vitamin D
(C) Vitamin D_2
(D) Vitamin D_3

9) Match the clinical manifestations on the left with the deficiency on the right.

1) Scaly dermatitis, alopecia, thrombocytopenia
2) Dry skin, poor wound healing, perioral rash
3) Hemolytic anemia, peripheral edema, thrombocytopenia

(A) Zinc deficiency
(B) Vitamin E deficiency
(C) Essential fatty acid deficiency
(D) Ascorbic acid deficiency

10) Regarding protocol in the *United States,* what would be the most appropriate nutrition to provide to a child born to a mother who is HIV-positive?

   A) Breast feeding
   B) Commercially prepared formula
   C) Filtered mother's breast milk
   D) Mother's breast milk after freezing[1]
   E) Pooled breast milk

11) Which of the following is TRUE regarding medium chain triglycerides?

   A) They are not present in human milk
   B) They are not present in cow's milk
   C) They are never present in commercially available infant formula
   D) They require micelle formation with bile salts for adequate absorption
   E) They are obtained by chopping triglycerides using a "medium-sized chain-saw"

12) Deficiency of biotin results in:

   A) Seborrhea
   B) Keratomalacia
   C) Glossitis
   D) Oxaluria
   E) Sensory neuropathy

13) Oxaluria would *most likely* be the result of the EXCESS of which of the following?

   A) Niacin
   B) Ascorbic acid
   C) Riboflavin
   D) Cyanocobalamin
   E) Retinol

---

[1] Freezing the milk, not the mother or her breast.

14) An adolescent girl following a strict vegan diet is most likely to develop deficiency of which of the following water-soluble vitamins?

A) Folic acid
B) Niacin
C) Riboflavin
D) Cobalamin
E) Thiamine

15) You are evaluating a 6 year old child recently adopted from China. The parents are very concerned because the child seems to bump into objects in the evening after he has completed his homework and is getting ready for bed.

The teachers state that he has no similar difficulty at school. He is below the 25th percentile for weight and height. On physical examination he is noted to have skin which is dry and scaly. In addition, silver patches are noted on his conjunctiva. What is the most likely explanation for the child's clinical presentation?

A) Tocopherol deficiency
B) Attention deficit hyperactivity disorder
C) Retinol deficiency
D) Chronic use of methylphenidate
E) Psoriasis

16) You are asked to evaluate a 9 month old white male who has been breast fed exclusively. He has had recurrent episodes of bronchiolitis and foul smelling diarrhea.

On physical exam the child appears small with decreased muscle tone. His conjunctiva are mildly injected. His labs findings include a low serum calcium, elevated alkaline phosphatase, and anemia with a slight increase in indirect bilirubin.

Which of the following would be the most likely explanation for *all* of the clinical findings?

A) Vitamin D deficiency
B) Vitamin E deficiency
C) Vitamin A deficiency
D) Poor exposure to UV light
E) Cystic fibrosis

17) You are evaluating a one week old boy who is visiting from out of town. He has been exclusively breast-fed. You note mild bleeding from the nares, the umbilical stump and the circumcision site. The infant has not been seen by his pediatrician or any other clinician other than the nurse midwife who delivered the baby at home.

The most appropriate treatment of this baby will be:

A) Vitamin K
B) Fresh frozen plasma
C) Van Willebrand Factor
D) Factor 8
E) Factor 9

18) Which of the following is true regarding the caloric needs of full term vs. preterm infants?

A) Full term infants require 100- 120 Kcal / Kg / day
B) Preterm infants require 100- 120 Kcal/ Kg/ day
C) A and B
D) Full term infants require a minimum 150 Kcal/Kg/day
E) Preterm infants require 80-100 Kcal/Kg/ day

19) You are managing a severely malnourished 16 year old female admitted for management of anorexia nervosa. She must be medically cleared before receiving psychiatric treatment. During refeeding, the most common electrolyte abnormality seen during the first week of treatment is:

A) Hyperphosphatemia
B) Hypophosphatemia
C) Hypocalcemia
D) Hypercalcemia
E) Hypernatremia

20) You are taking care of a one month old who has a documented gram negative sepsis. Additional findings include hepatomegaly, elevated indirect bilirubin and positive reducing substances in the stool.

The most likely explanation for this infant's clinical presentation would be:

A) Congenital toxoplasmosis infection
B) G6PD deficiency
C) Galactose-1-phosphate uridyltransferase deficiency
D) 21-hydroxylase deficiency
E) Congenital cytomegalovirus infection

Preventive Pediatrics

21) Regarding childhood drowning, each of the following is true EXCEPT:

A) It occurs more frequently in boys than girls
B) If swimming pools are excluded, those of lower socioeconomic status are at greater risk
C) Toddlers between the ages of 1 and 3 are at the greatest risk
D) Infant and toddler swimming lessons reduce the risk
E) A fence that surrounds and separates the pool from the house and yard significantly reduces the risk

22) You have been asked to give a talk to a group of new parents on preventing injuries. You are asked: "what is the most common way in which children receive burn injuries?" You correctly answer:

A) Matches
B) Fireplaces
C) Electrical wires
D) Hot liquids
E) Radiators

23) A 7-week-old infant in your practice develops a documented case of pertussis. The BEST treatment for his 6-1/2-year-old brother, who has received 5 doses of DTaP, the most recent one 2 years ago, would consist of:

   A) A DTaP booster and a 14-day course of rifampin
   B) No additional immunizations, but a 14-day course of erythromycin
   C) No additional immunizations, but a 14-day course of erythromycin at the start of any clinical sign
   D) No additional immunizations, but a 10-day course of rifampin
   E) A DTaP booster and a 5-day course of clarithromycin

24) All of the following are possible reactions to the varicella vaccine EXCEPT:

   A) Death
   B) Anaphylaxis
   C) Temporal lobe seizure
   D) Encephalitis
   E) ITP

25) Varicella vaccine is contraindicated in each of the following situations EXCEPT:

   A) Children with a history of an anaphylactic reaction to gelatin or neomycin
   B) Pregnant women
   C) Children receiving high-dose corticosteroids for more than 2 weeks
   D) HIV patients who are mildly symptomatic
   E) Children with acute lymphocytic leukemia who are not in remission

26) Which of the following is TRUE regarding cholesterol screening and promoting healthy cholesterol levels in children?

   A) Egg whites should be substituted for fats
   B) Total cholesterol or HDL levels require fasting
   C) Calculation of LDL cholesterol levels does not require fasting
   D) Cholesterol levels decrease before puberty and rapidly increase during the growth spurt.
   E) Changing to low-fat dairy products is sufficient for children younger than 2 years of age.

Poisons and Toxins

27) For accidental ingestion of which of the following would activated charcoal be most appropriate?

   A) Lithium carbonate
   B) Iron supplements
   C) Kerosene
   D) Beta Blockers
   E) Cyanide

28) You are managing a 2 year old patient who may have ingested a medication that her aunt uses for her upset stomach. You note a distinct wintergreen odor on her breath and suspect that she might have ingested an unknown amount of salicylate. Each of the following would be correct regarding the management of this patient except:

   A) Administer activated charcoal
   B) Obtain serum electrolytes
   C) Obtain acetaminophen level
   D) Initiate Gastric lavage
   E) Calculate the anion gap

29) You are presented with a toddler who was left alone in the garage for "just one second" and might have ingested an unknown amount of windshield wiper fluid. What is the best treatment option?

   A) Alkalization the urine
   B) Isopropyl alcohol as an alcohol dehydrogenase antagonist
   C) Ethyl alcohol (ethanol) as an alcohol dehydrogenase antagonist
   D) Hydroxocobalamin
   E) Gastric lavage

30) Which of the following is true regarding the ingestion of button batteries?

A) The highest morbidity is found with button batteries measuring 20 mm or smaller
B) It takes up to 24 hours before any serious burns can occur
C) Lithium based batteries are the least toxic
D) Button batteries that have passed into the stomach may be monitored with serial x-rays every 12 hours
E) Once the battery is removed, the degree of injury does not worsen

31) You are evaluating a 3-1/2 year old girl. On examination you notice that she is having a difficult time walking and seems less animated than usual when you offer her a sticker. Her blood pressure is 110/70, heart rate is 75 and she is afebrile. There is no history or signs of trauma and she is not taking any medication. However, she has had diarrhea over the past 2 days and the baby sitter might have given her some medication from the drug store for this. You note mild miosis. The diarrhea has been very mild and she has been drinking watered down sports drinks throughout the day without emesis. What is the most likely explanation for the presentation:

A) Severe dehydration
B) Loperamide ingestion
C) Hyperkalemia
D) Simethicone overdose
E) Hyponatremia

Fetus and Newborn

32) Which one of the following is a TRUE statement regarding *developmental dysplasia of the hip?* It is more common in:

   A) African-American babies
   B) Males
   C) SGA infants
   D) Premature infants
   E) Breech infants

33) You are called to the delivery room to see a newborn with herniation of the abdominal contents. You note that a membrane covers the bowel contents. Which of the following is TRUE regarding omphaloceles?

   A) They are a result of the failure of the umbilical ring to contract
   B) They are rarely associated with other anomalies
   C) They have been linked to a folate-deficient diet during pregnancy
   D) They have been associated with Beckwith-Wiedemann syndrome
   E) They may protrude through any defect in the abdominal wall

34) Each of the following newborn rashes requires nothing more than reassurance EXCEPT:

   A) Erythema toxicum
   B) Dry peeling skin
   C) Miliaria crystalline
   D) Midline lumbosacral skin tag
   E) Yellow papules on the hard palate

35) Despite attempts to halt labor, a 28-week premature baby boy is born while you are on-call. You are paged to the DR. The FIRST thing you should do after delivery is:

A) Assess respiratory status and prepare for intubation
B) Provide positive pressure ventilation
C) Place infant on an open bed warmer as a source of radiant heat
D) Place oxygen saturation monitor on your finger tip with the alarm set for a saturation below 55% and a pulse greater than 375
E) Obtain oxygen saturation monitor reading and establish an airway

36) Much has been written about maternal-baby bonding. There have been an equal number of super bowl infomercials on male bonding and recent emphasis on father-infant bonding. The MOST important factor in predicting father child bonding is:

A) The number of children the father has had
B) Whether the diaper genie is shaped like one of the "Bud Bowl" players
C) How many times the father has watched the Dr. Phil show
D) The age of the father
E) The father's presence in the delivery room

37) A 5-week-old first-born male is presented to you with a history of projectile vomiting of increasing severity. The baby looks dehydrated and hungry. You palpate an olive on the abdominal exam, and the father, who happens to be a surgeon, notes that he felt the "pit" in the olive. Prior to making your brilliant diagnosis of pyloric stenosis, which will be confirmed on ultrasound, the lab values you will MOST LIKELY have to correct are:

A) Sodium 145, potassium 3.7, bicarb 24, chloride 100
B) Sodium 138, potassium 3.0, bicarb 35, chloride 87
C) Sodium 134, potassium 6.0, bicarb 20, chloride 90
D) Sodium 140, potassium 3.3, bicarb 25, chloride 108
E) Sodium 150, potassium 5.2, bicarb 10, chloride 124

QUESTIONS: Fetus and Newborn

38) Which of the following statements regarding pyloric stenosis is true?

   A) It occurs more frequently in females
   B) It results in a hyperchloremic metabolic alkalosis
   C) A skilled pediatrician can palpate the "olive" 95% of the time but only a skilled surgeon can feel the "pimento" in the olive
   D) Post-op apnea is best prevented through pre-op rehydration and correction of metabolic alkalosis
   E) The family history on the father's side is usually positive

39) An infant is born to a mother who was treated for eclampsia. The Apgar scores were low, and the neonate is noted to have poor tone with decreased deep tendon reflexes and lethargy. The *most likely* cause is:

   A) Hypoglycemia
   B) Hypocalcemia
   C) Hypernatremia
   D) Hypermanganesemia
   E) Hypermagnesemia

40) At the routine 2-week visit, an infant is noted to have left-sided tilting of the head and a firm mass in the sternomastoid muscle on the left side. The *most appropriate* next step in the management would be:

   A) Have the baby do the hokie pokie and turn his head around
   B) Biopsy of the nodule
   C) MRI of the head
   D) EMG
   E) Passive stretching exercise

41) A former ventilator-dependent premie with bronchopulmonary dysplasia (BPD) is admitted for a hernia repair. His routine medications include furosemide and potassium chloride supplements. You obtain an arterial blood gas and, with the infant on 40% oxygen, the results of the ABG are pH 7.49, PCO_2 55 mm Hg, and PO_2 90 mm HG. These findings are *best* explained by:

A) Nephrocalcinosis
B) Primary respiratory alkalosis
C) Furosemide-induced alkalosis
D) Appropriate for an infant with BPD
E) Most likely a result of lab error

42) A 4-month-old infant is referred to you by a family practitioner because of a bulging fontanelle and poor feeding.[2] The infant's parents insist on feeding "natural foods" and the "natural doctor" suggested they feed the infant large amounts of natural vitamin and mineral supplements, which they have done for over 3 weeks. An excess of which of the following would be *most likely* to cause the patient's symptoms?

A) Vitamin C
B) Manganese
C) Vitamin D
D) Zinc
E) Vitamin A

43) A newborn, born at 36 weeks gestation via an uneventful spontaneous vaginal delivery, develops progressive respiratory distress with cyanosis. Chest x-ray is remarkable for cardiomegaly as well as diffuse granular pattern and bilateral pleural effusions. At 3 hours of age, hypotension develops. The CBC is unremarkable. Which of the following is the *most likely* cause of this infant's respiratory problem?

A) Total anomalous pulmonary venous connection
B) Transient tachypnea of the newborn
C) Group B *Strep* pneumonia
D) Respiratory Distress Sydrome
E) Meconium aspiration syndrome

---

[2] We're talking about the infant; the referring physician is fine.

QUESTIONS: Fetus and Newborn

44) You are evaluating a full term 3.6 kg infant born by repeat C/Section. The apgar scores were 7/9 and the respiratory rate is 80 with a heart rate of 160. The oxygen saturations dip to the low 90s on room air and the baby is given supplemental oxygen. On the physical exam you note some mild subcostal retractions with good air movement. There are no cardiac murmurs noted. You order a CXR which reveals increased interstitial markings and fluid in some of the interlobar fissures.

    The most likely diagnosis is:

    A) Tetralogy of Fallot
    B) Respiratory distress syndrome
    C) Group B Strep pneumonia
    D) Transient tachypnea of the newborn
    E) Pulmonary hypertension

45) Approximately what percentage of newborns require some form of resuscitation in the delivery room?

    A) 1%
    B) 10%
    C) 25%
    D) 50%
    E) 65%

46) Within the first hour post delivery, which of the following should receive top priority?

    A) Vitamin K IM
    B) Erythromycin ophthalmic ointment
    C) Obtaining a weight
    D) Measuring length
    E) Allowing the infant to breast feed

47) Discharge from the newborn nursery after a normal spontaneous vaginal delivery is considered "early" when it's prior to:

A) 12 hours
B) 24 hours
C) 48 hours
D) 72 hours
E) Depends on the HMO the parent's are enrolled in

48) Infants must be seen within 48 hours if they are discharged prior to:

A) 12 hours
B) 24 hours
C) 48 hours
D) 72 hours
E) Depends on the pediatrician

49) Breastfeeding jaundice commonly seen in the first 2-4 postnatal days is due to:

A) Decreased bilirubin conjugation
B) Decreased ligandin
C) IgA present in breast milk
D) Increased entero-hepatic circulation
E) Decreased entero-hepatic circulation

50) You are evaluating a 6 week old infant who is breastfeeding well and having 3-4 clay colored stools per day. On physical examination, the baby is icteric with jaundice to the pelvic area.

The most likely explanation for the presentation is:

A) Breast feeding jaundice
B) Human milk associated jaundice
C) Cholestasis
D) Gilbert Syndrome
E) ABO incompatibility

QUESTIONS: Fetus and Newborn

51) Which of the following is true regarding conjugated hyperbilirubinemia?

   A) It is the exact same thing as direct hyperbilirubinemia
   B) It is always associated with cholestasis
   C) It is more common than unconjugated hyperbilirubinemia
   D) It is defined as conjugated bilirubin greater than 2.0 or greater than 20% of the total bilirubin
   E) It is seen in Gilbert syndrome

52) You are evaluating a full-term infant that presents with noisy breathing and copious secretions requiring repeated suctioning from the oropharynx. The initial glucose water feeding results in a severe choking episode. The MOST appropriate next step would be to:

   A) Ask the most experienced nurse to feed the infant and report results
   B) Request a barium swallow examination
   C) Obtain a CT of the head immediately
   D) Insert a catheter into both nares to assure patency
   E) Obtain an x-ray study of the chest after inserting a soft radiopaque feeding tube

53) In addition to premature closure of the ductus arteriosus, the fetus exposed to indomethacin would have all the additional adverse effects EXCEPT:

   A) Irreversible renal failure
   B) Oligohydramnios
   C) Increased risk for periventricular leukomalacia
   D) Increased risk for necrotizing enterocolitis
   E) Reversible renal failure

54) Each of the following is true and/or associated with gastroesophageal reflux in infants *except:*

   A) Chronic wheezing
   B) Failure to thrive
   C) Head elevation in the supine position is always helpful
   D) Regurgitation often occurs 30 minutes after feeding
   E) Irritability during or after feedings

55) Each of the following is true of, or associated with, rumination in infants *except*:

   A) Repeated and painless regurgitation
   B) Symptoms do not occur during sleep
   C) It does not respond to standard treatment for gastroesophageal reflux
   D) Symptoms must be present for 8 weeks or longer
   E) It is associated with retching

Fluids and Lytes

56) The molar ratio of glucose to sodium in standard oral rehydration solution should not exceed:

   A) 3:1
   B) 2:1
   C) 1:1
   D) 1:3
   E) Molar? This isn't the dental boards! C'mon

57) An 8 week old boy is brought to you in the ER by a panic stricken mother after he has had a generalized seizure. He has had some pretty bad diarrhea according to the mother. You find out that besides breast milk, the *grandmother* has done what she has always done in such cases and gave the baby lots of diluted tea. You order Lytes superstat and are shocked and horrified to find a serum sodium of 110. Your next step is to:

   A) Find out more about the tea that packs that kind of punch
   B) Order NS 20 cc/KG over 15 – 20 minutes, repeated until clinically warranted
   C) Order NS IV maintenance, half over the next 8 hours and the other half over 16 hours
   D) Order a 3% saline solution bolus 5 – 6 ml/kg over a few minutes
   E) Order a 0.3% saline solution bolus 5 – 6 ml/kg over a few minutes

QUESTIONS: Fluids and Lytes

58) You are caring for an infant diagnosed with hypernatremic dehydration. It is December and you have been a PGY1 for close to 6 months now. You have seen one, done one, taught one, 300 times now, but who is counting. The chief resident, along with the rest of the residents, decides to go to the holiday party and you are left to fend for yourself. This child is in good hands because you know that he is at risk for developing a seizure due to :

A) Central pontine myelinolysis
B) The shifting of extra cellular and interstitial fluids
C) Rapid change in sodium concentration
D) Rapid change in glucose concentration
E) Rapid change in the blood ethanol alcohol of the rest of the house staff attending the party

59) An 18-month-old has a one-week history of vomiting and diarrhea. His grandmother has given him a rice, water, and salt mixture. He appears lethargic and irritable and has doughy abdominal skin.[3] Which of the following lab results would BEST explain the findings?

A) Serum chloride concentration of 97 mEq/L
B) Blood glucose concentration of 95 mg/dL
C) Blood glucose concentration of 170 mg/dL
D) Serum sodium concentration of 125 mEq/L
E) Serum sodium concentration of 165 mEq/L

60) Each of the following is associated with hemolytic uremic syndrome (HUS) EXCEPT:

A) Hyponatremia
B) Hypokalemia
C) Metabolic acidosis
D) Hyperphosphatemia
E) Thrombocytopenia

---

[3] Not unlike the doughy abdominal skin of the average person studying for the boards.

61) A child with asthma is examined during an episode that has lasted for a few hours. Except for tachypnea, wheezing, and retractions, there are no abnormal findings on physical examination.

ABG reveals a pH of 7.25, PCO_2 of 30, and PO_2 of 70. The probable cause of the acidemia is:

A) Respiratory owing to CO_2 retention
B) Metabolic owing to renal compensation
C) Metabolic owing to reduced cardiac output
D) Respiratory owing to excessive CO_2 loss
E) Metabolic owing to poor tissue oxygenation

62) In the face of hypernatremia, in order to maintain homeostasis, idiogenic osmoles are produced in which of the following tissues:

A) Testicular
B) Renal
C) Spleen
D) Central Nervous System
E) Both A and D

63) Which of the following would be commonly seen in Cushing Syndrome?

A) Edema
B) Hypertension
C) Decreased body weight
D) Hypernatremia
E) Hyponatremia

64) Each of the following would cause a respiratory alkalosis *except* for:

   A) Pneumonia
   B) Asthma
   C) Salicylate toxicity
   D) Barbiturate toxicity
   E) Pulmonary edema

65) Respiratory acidosis may result from each of the following except:

   A) Spinal cord injury
   B) Myasthenia crisis
   C) Guillain-Barré syndrome
   D) Nicotine toxicity
   E) Botulism

66) Each of the following is an adverse consequences of severe acidemia *except:*

   A) Hyperventilation
   B) Dyspnea
   C) Arteriole dilation
   D) Enhanced cardiac contractility
   E) Insulin resistance

67) Each of the following may lead to metabolic acidosis with a normal anion gap except:

   A) Diarrhea
   B) Pancreatic fistula
   C) Hypoaldosteronism
   D) Ethylene glycol ingestion
   E) Renal tubular acidosis.

Genetics

68) Each of the following is true regarding Down syndrome (Trisomy 21) EXCEPT:

A) The risk for transmission is higher if the mother is the carrier of a balanced translocation
B) Children with Down syndrome due to a parental translocation are phenotypically different from those due to standard trisomy
C) Mothers in their 20s have more children with Down syndrome than any other age group
D) If the mother has a translocation, the risk of recurrence is 14%
E) In the absence of translocation, the risk of recurrence is 1%

69) An 8-year-old boy diagnosed with intellectual disability[4] is sent for genetic studies. DNA analysis reveals an expanded segment of the CGG segment of DNA in the q27 region of the X chromosome. Which of the following will most likely be found in this patient at puberty?

A) An accelerated growth spurt
B) Macroorchidism
C) Breast enlargement
D) Further deterioration of intellect
E) Progressive myopathy

70) You are called upon by a couple who have 2 children with Lesch-Nyhan syndrome and a 12-year-old boy who is unaffected by the disease. The parents call you at 3AM because they can't sleep and to find out the chances of their 12-year-old son having an affected child of his own when he starts a family in the distant future.

Now you can't sleep either. You turn on your night light, remove the crust from your eyes, and tell them:

Since Lesch-Nyhan syndrome is inherited in an X-linked recessive manner, you fall back to sleep while the parents are still speaking with you. They call you back and you tell them that the risk for the unaffected brother having a child with Lesch-Nyhan syndrome is:

A) No greater than that of any person in the general population regardless of gender.
B) 25% regardless of gender
C) 50% if the child is a girl and 0% if the child is a boy
D) 50% if the child is a boy and 0% if the child is a girl
E) Much lower if they had been considerate enough to call you during regular office hours

---

[4] The term intellectual disability has replaced the term mental retardation. President Obama actually signed a bill in October 2010 making this official.

QUESTIONS: Genetics

71) Each of the following is associated with Cri-du – Chat syndrome EXCEPT:

A) Macrocephaly
B) Epicanthal folds
C) Cardiac defects
D) Cat like cry
E) Psychomotor retardation

72) Each of the following is associated with Russel Silver syndrome EXCEPT:

A) Cardiac defects
B) Abnormalities in the 5th finger
C) Triangle face
D) Wide spaced teeth
E) Normal head circumference

73) You are evaluating an infant with a hairy back. Long curly eyebrows, long philtrum, wide spaced teeth, hearing loss and a small head. The most likely diagnosis is:

A) Rubinstein Taybi Syndrome
B) Russel Silver Syndrome
C) Cornelia de Lange Syndrome
D) Contestant on American Idol
E) Noonan syndrome

74) You are evaluating a child with macroglossia, hemihypertrophy, cardiomegaly, and hepatomegaly. The most likely diagnosis is:

A) Wilms tumor
B) Noonan Syndrome
C) Russel Silver Syndrome
D) Rubinstein Taybi Syndrome
E) Beckwith-Wiedemann Syndrome

75) You are evaluating a patient with broad thumbs and great toes, as well as a beaked nose, and cardiac abnormalities.

The most likely diagnosis is:

A) Noonan syndrome
B) Russel Silver Syndrome
C) Rubinstein Taybi Syndrome
D) Beckwith Wiedemann Syndrome.
E) Pierre Robin Syndrome

76) Each of the following is associated with Klinefelter syndrome EXCEPT:

A) Increased risk for breast cancer
B) Testosterone replacement therapy
C) XYY Karyotype
D) Intellectual ability *slightly* below the general population
E) Leading cause of male infertility

77) Which of the following medications are considered to be safe during pregnancy?

A) Warfarin
B) Heparin
C) ACE inhibitors
D) Valproic Acid
E) Carbamazepine

78) You are evaluating a newborn who has deviation of the nose to one side, feet that remain medially rotated, and the right outer ear folded down.

The most likely explanation would be:

A) Gestational diabetes
B) Eclampsia
C) Anticonvulsant exposure
D) Oligohydramnios
E) Fetal alcohol syndrome

QUESTIONS: Genetics

79) A boy in your practice is born with a tracheoesophageal fistula (TEF) with no other abnormal physical findings. The parents are concerned about the possibility of conceiving another child with the same problem. The correct answer would be:

   A) Boys have a 50% chance
   B) The same chance as in the general population
   C) 25% regardless of gender
   D) 4% regardless of gender
   E) Girls have a 50% chance

80) You are evaluating an infant born with a persistent patent ductus arteriosis and documented fetal anuria.

   Exposure to which of the following medications would BEST explain this combination of findings.

   A) Serotonin reuptake inhibitors
   B) Heparin
   C) Warfarin
   D) Phenytoin
   E) ACE inhibitors

81) Exposure to which of the following best explains an infant born with an atrial septal defect and thyroid disturbances.

   A) ACE inhibitors
   B) Heparin
   C) Serotonin reuptake inhibitors
   D) Lithium
   E) Acetaminophen

Allergy and Immunology

82) Match the immune response description on the left with the classified allergic reaction on the right.

    1) Immune complex (Arthus reaction)   (A) Type 1 allergic reaction
    2) Delayed hypersensitivity   (B) Type 2 allergic reaction
    3) Anaphylactoid reaction   (C) Type 3 allergic reaction
    4) Antibody mediated   (D) Type 4 allergic reaction

83) It's a Friday afternoon, the snow is blowing and the sun is setting, and you're thinking about the skiing trip you are headed for. "Doctor, we have a drop in: 7 year old Sammy Snowster. He has fever and an earache." You glance at the problem list:

It's his ninth ear infection and each time he has had symptoms consistent with sinusitis.

In addition, he has had multiple episodes of bronchitis.

His immunizations are all up to date.

His physical exam is unremarkable except for the "I'm with Stupid" shirt he is wearing with the arrow pointed in your direction.

His CBC, electrolytes and liver function tests have been consistently normal.

Your partner did check his hepatitis B titers, which were significantly low for someone who had completed his immunization set. You scratch your head, move out of the way so the arrow isn't pointed at you, and redeem yourself by making the following diagnosis:

A) Poor wardrobe. You replace his shirt with one that says "Don't Mess with Mr. Zero."
B) Just a poor response to the hepatitis B vaccine. After another full series, there should be no problem.
C) X-linked severe immunodeficiency.
D) Common variable immunodeficiency.
E) HIV. You start Bactrim prophylaxis and begin a full workup.

QUESTIONS: Allergy and Immunology

84) **A 6-month-old exclusively breast fed infant presents with a diffuse dry patchy, scaly erythematous skin rash worse on extensor surfaces. Itching is relieved partially with twice daily diphenhydramine. The MOST appropriate next step would be to:**

A) Switch to a soy based formula
B) Skin test the baby
C) Skin test the mother
D) Start oral steroids
E) Order IgE levels on the baby

85) **The most common primary immunodeficiency is:**

A) Chronic granulomatous disease
B) AIDS
C) Selective IgA deficiency
D) Congenital X-linked agammaglobulinemia
E) Hyperimmunoglobulin E syndrome

86) **You are managing a patient in your practice who presents with failure to thrive, chronic diarrhea and candidal infections resistant to treatment. Lab results reveal hypocalcemia. Genetic studies reveal a hemizygous deletion of 22q11.2**

Which of the following options would be most appropriate in this patient?

A) Splenectomy
B) Bone marrow transplantation
C) Monthly T-lymphocyte replacement
D) Thymectomy
E) Thymic transplantation

87) Each of the following is true regarding X-linked hyper IgM syndrome EXCEPT:

   A) Prophylaxis against P. jiroveci is indicated
   B) Intravenous gammaglobulin treatment is indicated
   C) IgG, IgA, IgE levels are low
   D) IgM levels are elevated
   E) IgG, IgA and IgE levels are elevated

88) Which of the following is true regarding IgA deficiency?

   A) It is the least common primary immunodeficiency
   B) Most patients with this defect have recurrent infections.
   C) IgA deficiency is an indication for replacement immunoglobulin therapy
   D) Circulating anti-IgA antibodies places patients at risk if transfused with immunoglobulin
   E) Most asymptomatic cases have defects in one or more IgG subclasses

89) Which of the following is true regarding the use of inhaled steroids in treating asthma?

   A) They are risk-free
   B) On average, final adult height is 0.5 cm below expected
   C) Growth velocity is reduced during the first year of treatment
   D) Acne, mood swings and weight gain do not occur
   E) Oral candidiasis is a rare complication

90) Which of the following is the most appropriate treatment of chronic urticaria?

   A) Topical diphenhydramine
   B) Topical hydrocortisone 2% lotion
   C) Hydroxyzine
   D) Diphenhydramine
   E) Fexofenadine

Infectious Disease

91) A 2 year old child presents to your office with a history of fever spikes of 104 degrees with cough, coryza, and conjunctivitis. You brilliantly diagnose measles – something that still occurs, mostly on the boards. Which of the following is correct with regards to measles?

   A) Elevated measles specific IgM at presentation is diagnostic
   B) Good hand washing prevents spread of disease
   C) Patients are contagious from 2 days before becoming symptomatic until 4 days after the onset of the rash
   D) No need to know anything about this measly disease since there is a vaccine
   E) Acute encephalitis is a common complication

92) During an outbreak of measles, vaccination would be indicated for each of the following EXCEPT for:

   A) A unimmunized 3 year old exposed 2 days earlier
   B) An unimmunized 12 month old exposed 2 days earlier
   C) A symptomatic HIV patient
   D) A 5 year old, who is HIV positive with high CD4 T lymphocyte count, exposed 24 hours earlier
   E) A nonimmune pregnant woman exposed 2 days ago

93) All of the following are true about rubella EXCEPT:

   A) It is an illness with high morbidity that presents with high fever and an erythematous rash
   B) During the pre-vaccine era, inapparent infection was common
   C) The period of communicability begins 2 days before the appearance of the rash and lasts another 7 days
   D) Infants with congenital rubella should be considered contagious until they are 1 year old or get a confirmed negative by repeat culture
   E) Children with rubella are considered contagious for 1 year or the beginning of Oktoberfest, whichever occurs first

94) Confirmed cases of active pulmonary tuberculosis are treated with which of the following?

   A) Ethambutol
   B) Pyrazinamide
   C) Rifampin
   D) Isoniazid
   E) B, C, and D

95) You suspect a child has active tuberculosis, yet his skin test is negative. You remember that false negatives can occur in each of the following situations EXCEPT:

   A) The child has only recently been infected but has not developed sensitivity yet
   B) The child has had a recent viral infection
   C) Poor technique was used
   D) Kwashiorkor coexists
   E) The child received prior vaccination with BCG

96) The *most appropriate* treatment for the cat bite above would be:

   A) Observation and conservative management
   B) Intravenous cefazolin
   C) Oral amoxicillin/clavulanic acid
   D) Oral penicillin
   E) IV penicillin

97) Of the following, the *most specific* diagnostic test for acute herpes simplex virus infection is:

   A) An enzyme immunoassay
   B) Isolation of the virus by a culture
   C) Identification of giant multinucleated cells on a Tzanck smear
   D) The development of specific neutralizing antibodies
   E) Serum IgM

QUESTIONS: Infectious Disease

98) A 6-year-old girl has had varicella for four days. Several of the lesions on her abdomen have developed honey-colored crusts, purulent exudate, and surrounding cellulitis. Gram stain reveals gram-positive cocci in clusters. Which of the following is the MOST appropriate initial treatment?

A) Cefazolin
B) Trimethoprim with sulfamethoxazole
C) Tetracycline
D) Acyclovir
E) Rifampin

99) A 1-month-old infant presents with irritability and poor feeding. Temperature is 40 C. On physical examination you note that the infant is responsive but markedly irritable, with a left tympanic membrane that is bulging and erythematous. The right tympanic membrane is clear. After obtaining the appropriate lab studies, the MOST appropriate antibiotic treatment would consist of:

A) Ampicillin
B) Cefoxitin
C) Cefotaxime
D) Oral amoxicillin with close followup
E) Ampicillin and gentamicin

100) A 4-year-old girl with a 4-day history of fever is admitted to your service. She has had bloody diarrhea for over a week coupled with decreased urinary output.

On physical examination, you note that she is pale and has some edema. CBC is remarkable for a low hematocrit and platelet count. The WBC is normal. Fragmented red cells are noted on the peripheral smear. Urinalysis is positive for blood and the BUN is 75 with a creatinine of 2.9. Your admitting diagnosis is:

A) *Salmonella* diarrhea and sepsis
B) Henoch-Schönlein purpura
C) Shigella
D) Toxic shock syndrome
E) Hemolytic uremic syndrome

101) A 10-week-old infant presents with a 3-day history of a staccato cough. The infant is in mild respiratory distress and is afebrile with stable vital signs.

A CBC reveals a WBC of 12.5 with 22% polys, 5% bands, 65% lymphocytes, and 7% eosinophils. Chest x-ray shows no focal infiltrates, but is remarkable for *diffuse* infiltrates with some hyperinflation. You'd be correct in treating with:

A) IV cefuroxime
B) PO erythromycin
C) Albuterol nebulized treatments
D) High dose corticosteroids
E) Observation

102) A 6-month-old child is diagnosed with pertussis. Each of the following is true regarding azithromycin prophylaxis EXCEPT:

A) It would be indicated for the infant's father
B) It would be indicated for the infant's 3-year-old sibling only if he is unimmunized
C) It would be indicated for the infant's 5-year-old sibling regardless of immunization status
D) It would be indicated in the infant's caretaker at the childcare center
E) It would be indicated for the grandmother living with the family

103) Which of the following antibiotics should be avoided in patients with known neuromuscular disease?

A) Ampicillin
B) Gentamicin
C) Metronidazole
D) Ceftriaxone
E) Vancomycin
F) None of the above

QUESTIONS: Infectious Disease

104) Infection with each of the following can mimic Epstein-Barr (EBV) infectious mononucleosis EXCEPT:

   A) Cytomegalovirus
   B) Adenovirus
   C) Human herpes virus (HHV) – 6
   D) Paramyxovirus
   E) Rubella

105) The medical and housekeeping staff liked your presentations so much, they have asked you to give a noon conference on safety precautions and infection control in the office setting. Each of the following is true regarding the handling of sharps in an office practice EXCEPT:

   A) Do not recap the needles using two hands
   B) Discard sharps yourself, even if an assistant is close by with closer access to the container
   C) Discard sharps immediately after use in a nearby designated container
   D) Discard the sharps container as soon as it is full
   E) Make the sharp contents accessible to the staff but inaccessible to patients

106) Which of the following is the most common cutaneous manifestation of secondary syphilis?

   A) Condylomata lata
   B) Non-pruritic palmar maculopapules
   C) Mocha latte
   D) Palmar vesiculopustules
   E) Emerson, Lake, and Palmar

107) Sensorineural hearing loss resulting from direct invasion of the inner ear is the most common manifestation of which of the following viral infections?

   A) Congenital CMV
   B) Congenital HSV
   C) Influenza
   D) Rubeola
   E) Coxsackie

108) Which of the following complications of disseminated gonococcal infection would be likely in an adolescent girl?

A) Meningitis
B) Hepatitis
C) Osteomyelitis
D) Perihepatitis
E) Endocarditis

109) Waiting in your previously neat reception area are 50 to 100 students who recently helped clean up a park in Indiana. They all recently developed an influenza-like syndrome including a low-grade fever, muscular aches, crackles on chest auscultation, hepatosplenomegaly and decreased appetite. The symptoms are probably a result of:

A) Influenza
B) Cryptococcosis
C) Aspergillosis
D) Histoplasmosis
E) Hardus workus shockus

110) A one month old is anemic, irritable, and noted to have skin lesions on the palms and soles. On physical examination, you also note hepatosplenomegaly and decreased movement of the extremities. Which of the following is the *most likely* diagnosis?

A) Gonorrhea
B) Syphilis
C) Group B streptococcal infection
D) Cytomegalovirus infection
E) Toxoplasmosis

QUESTIONS: Infectious Disease

111) You are evaluating an 8 year old boy who presents with fever, cough and malaise for 5 days. Chest x-ray shows bilateral diffuse infiltrates.

The best treatment for this patient would be?

A) Supportive care including antipyretics
B) Supportive care including antipyretics and dextromethorphan
C) Azithromycin
D) Amoxicillin
E) Amoxicillin/clavulanic acid

112) Which of the following antibiotics would be the *best* choice in a 7 year old being treated with high dose amoxicillin for otitis media who is still symptomatic after 3 days of treatment and has a bulging erythematous tympanic membrane which does not move with insufflation?

A) Azithromycin
B) Higher dose amoxicillin
C) Amoxicillin clavulanic acid
D) Ciprofloxacin
E) Tetracycline

113) Each of the following antibiotics would be appropriate initial treatment in a patient suspected of having a skin infections caused by community acquired methicillin resistant Staph aureus *except:*

A) Amoxicillin/ clavulanic acid
B) Clindamycin
C) Trimethoprim/sulfamethoxazole
D) Linezolid
E) Vancomycin

114) Each of the following could be *a part of* prophylaxis for a male resident who examined the throat of a patient with a confirmed diagnosis of meningococcal sepsis (Serogroup A) *except?*

   A) Rifampin 600 mg BID for 2 days
   B) Rifampin 1200 mg q day for 4 days
   C) Ceftriaxone 250 mg IM once
   D) Ciprofloxacin 500 mg PO x 1
   E) Meningococcal vaccine

115) Which of the following is true regarding *Listeria monocytogenes* infection?

   A) Mothers of affected infants are always asymptomatic prior to delivery
   B) Listerosis typically presents with monocytosis
   C) The most common mode of transmission in mothers is via contaminated food
   D) Listerosis typically presents with monocytopenia
   E) Listeriosis typically presents with leukopenia

116) In addition to gentamicin, which of the following would be most appropriate to be used in a patient with *Listeria monocytogenes* meningitis who is allergic to penicillin?

   A) Cefotaxime
   B) Ceftriaxone
   C) Trimethoprim-sulfamethoxazole
   D) Chloramphenicol
   E) Ampicillin

117) You are caring for a child with cat scratch disease (CSD). The child is otherwise healthy with normal growth and development, his immunizations up to date and he has no past history of recurrent infections. Which of the following is the most appropriate management?

   A) Lymph node biopsy
   B) Amoxicillin / clavulanic acid
   C) Prednisone
   D) Cephalexin
   E) Supportive care and observation

QUESTIONS: Infectious Disease

118) All of the following are true regarding the incubation period following a bite by a rabies infected animal *except:*

   A) Incubation periods are longer in children
   B) Incubation period are shorter in those on chronic steroids
   C) Incubation periods are shorter with bites closer to the CNS
   D) The mean incubation period is 30-90 days
   E) A higher number of bites shortens the incubation period

119) You are presented with a patient whose HBsAg, is positive but the HBcAb and HBsAb are both negative. What is the correct interpretation of these results?

   A) Beam me up Scotty I have one for Mr. Spock
   B) Immune after hepatitis B vaccination
   C) Cannot tell if there is active disease without HbeAb status
   D) Active hepatitis B infection
   E) Immune after recovery from hepatitis B infection

120) Which of the following positive results is associated with a high hepatitis B viral replication rate?

   A) HBeAb
   B) HBeAg
   C) HBsAb
   D) HBsAg
   E) Helpmyeyesaresoglazedovermothshavebeenlandingonmyeyeswithoutmynoticing

121) Which of the following is associated with immunity following recovery form hepatitis B natural infection?

   A) HBeAb
   B) HBeAg
   C) HBcAb
   D) HBcAg
   E) HowtheheckshouldIknow?

Inborn Errors of Metabolism

122) All of the following are autosomal recessive disorders *EXCEPT*:

   A) Hunters syndrome
   B) Hurlers syndrome
   C) Tay Sachs disease
   D) Wilson's disease
   E) Kartagener's syndrome

123) In the following set of questions, decide if each numbered choice applies to (A) only, (B) only, both (C), or neither (D):

   1) Coarse facies
   2) Corneal clouding
   3) Autosomal recessive
   4) X-linked recessive
   5) Skeletal involvement/ normal intelligence

   (A) Hunters syndrome
   (B) Hurlers syndrome
   (C) Both
   (D) Neither

124) A 6-month-old infant presents with developmental delay. The prenatal and delivery histories are both unremarkable. Initial development was normal.

   However, the patient still has poor head control and the mother says he feels like "a jelly fish" without the container. The mother reports that the urine has taken on an odd odor and the initial hair was dark and is now much lighter. In addition to hypotonia, the physical exam is remarkable for weight in the 5%ile for age. Of the following, the most likely diagnosis in this clinical situation is:

   A) Tyrosinase negative albinism
   B) Galactosemia
   C) Hereditary fructose intolerance
   D) Tay Sachs disease
   E) Phenylketonuria

QUESTIONS: Inborn Errors of Metabolism

125) Elevated serum ammonia levels would be seen with each of the following EXCEPT:

   A) Reye's syndrome
   B) Leigh disease
   C) Liver failure
   D) Methylmalonic academia
   E) Ornithine transcarbamoylase deficiency

126) A 3-year-old boy with mental retardation is noted to have choreoathetoid movements, hyperreflexia, spasticity of the left leg, and positive Babinski's sign. There are signs of self-mutilation of the fingers and buccal mucosa. Which of the following is the *most likely* associated metabolic abnormality?

   A) Increased BUN/Creatinine
   B) Intracranial calcification
   C) Increased urine organic acid concentration
   D) Hypoglycemia
   E) Increased serum uric acid concentration

127) You are evaluating a 4 month old baby because of generalized seizures. The infant has not gained weight or grown sufficiently. On physical examination you note hepatomegaly and a large abdomen in general. You note that the infant looks thin. Lab results are significant for hypoglycemia and elevated uric acid and lipid levels.

   The most likely diagnosis is:

   A) Von Gierke Disease
   B) Pompe disease
   C) Lesch-Nyhan syndrome
   D) Congenital CMV infection
   E) Congenital Toxoplasmosis

128) Which of the following is true regarding infants identified in newborn screening with elevated blood phenylalanine (PA) levels?

   A) All of them have PKU on further testing
   B) Most of them will have PKU
   C) Most of them won't have PKU
   D) Some will have biopterin deficiency
   E) C and D

129) A 5 month old full term infant with unremarkable birth history and normal newborn screening presents with constipation and eyelids which remain open and have to be closed manually. There is evidence of decreased tone on physical exam. The anterior fontanelle is of normal size. Otherwise growth and development have been normal. He has been taking his formula well and had recently started eating cereal.

   The most likely diagnosis is:

   A) Myasthenia gravis
   B) Hypothyroidism
   C) Mitochondrial disorder
   D) Botulism poisoning
   E) Glycogen storage disease

130) You are evaluating an adolescent who initially presented with tremors and anxiety. She now presents with hemolytic anemia and is icteric and with elevated PTT. Hepatomegaly is noted on physical exam.

   Measurement of which of the following is likely to reveal the correct diagnosis?

   A) Factor VIII levels
   B) Platelet count
   C) Liver function test
   D) Serum ceruloplasmin
   E) Indirect and direct bilirubin

Endocrinology

131) A newborn in your practice has a positive result on her newborn screen for hypothyroidism. Which of the following is the MOST appropriate *next* step in managing this patient?

   A) Obtain a serum Free T4 and TSH and begin treatment if hypothyroidism is confirmed
   B) Obtain a serum Free T4 and TSH and begin treatment immediately
   C) Check a thyroid binding globulin (TBG) level
   D) Check TSH at 2 weeks of age
   E) Send the infant for a repeat newborn screen.

132) Children who develop hypothyroidism after what age can expect to have no *permanent impairment* of intellectual or neurological function?

   A) 3 months
   B) 6 months
   C) 12 months
   D) 18 months
   E) 36 months

133) The most appropriate treatment for idiopathic central precocious puberty is:

   A) FSH
   B) LH
   C) Leuprolide
   D) Growth hormone
   E) GnRH

134) You are evaluating a 16 year old boy whose SMR is 2 and whose parents are concerned over his lack of pubertal development and being somewhat shorter than they would expect. His height was in the 60th percentile until age 12 and has gradually dropped to the 5th percentile. His weight remained in the 50th percentile. The boy's bone age is 14. The parents note that his older brother was also a "slow grower" The MOST likely explanation for the findings is:

A) Familial short stature
B) Constitutional growth delay
C) Hypothyroidism
D) Crohn Disease
E) Nutritional deficiency

135) You are evaluating a 16 year old boy who has dropped from the 50th to the 10th percentile for both weight and height since age 11. He otherwise feels fine. Which of following would be the most appropriate initial step in establishing the underlying cause for his growth failure?

A) Growth hormone level
B) Chromosomal analysis
C) Free T4 and TSH
D) Erythrocyte sedimentation rate
E) Serum cortisol levels

136) You suspect growth hormone deficiency as the underlying cause of short stature in a child. The most appropriate initial screen would be to order a:

A) Growth hormone level
B) GnRH level
C) Tissue transglutaminase antibody
D) IGF-1
E) Erythrocyte sedimentation level

QUESTIONS: Endocrinology

137) You suspect celiac disease to be the underlying cause of a child's short stature. You document a normal IgA concentration. The most appropriate initial screening test would be:

A) Erythrocyte sedimentation rate
B) Small bowel biopsy
C) Stool glutinoid binding mucosal binding protein
D) Tissue transglutaminase antibody level
E) Stool for reducing substances

138) You are evaluating a 17 year old girl who has been complaining of gradually increasing headaches and visual deficits. Despite an SMR of 4 she has not started to menstruate. The most appropriate blood test to order would be a serum:

A) TSH
B) GnRH
C) LH
D) Prolactin
E) IGF-1:

139) The family of an 8-year-old boy expresses concern about his growth. Past records reveal that the child has been healthy and that height and weight have consistently been at the 5%ile. The father's height is 163 cm (64 inches) and the mother's is 152 cm (60 in). Physical examination reveals a healthy, prepubertal boy. The bone age is 8. Which of the following patterns is MOST likely in this child?

	Adult Stature	Pubertal Onset	Rate of Progression
A)	3%ile	Normal	Normal
B)	25%ile	Delayed	Slow
C)	50%ile	Early	Rapid
D)	50%ile	Early	Slow
E)	50%ile	Normal	Normal

140) You are evaluating a 2 year old who is walking bow legged, and whose ankles and wrists seem to be enlarged and there are bumps along his rib cage. He is below the 25th percentile for height and weight. CBC and ESR are within normal limits. Parathyroid hormone, 1, 25 Vitamin D, 25, Vitamin D, and calcium levels are all within normal limits. His alkaline phosphatase levels are markedly elevated and serum phosphate levels are well below normal.

The most likely explanation for these findings is

A) Nutritional neglect
B) Physical abuse
C) Vitamin D dependent rickets Type 1
D) Vitamin D Resistant Rickets
E) Familial hypophosphatemic rickets

141) You are evaluating a 2 year old African American lactose intolerant child who is walking bow legged, and whose ankles and wrists seem to be enlarged and there are bumps along his rib cage. The CBC and ESR are within normal limits. 25-Vitamin D, serum phosphate and calcium are all low. Alkaline phosphate and PTH are high.

The most likely explanation for these findings is

A) Vitamin D deficient rickets
B) Vitamin D dependent rickets Type 1
C) Vitamin D resistant Rickets
D) X- Linked hypophosphatemic rickets
E) Hypophosphatasia

142) You are evaluating a 2 year old who is walking bow legged, and whose ankles and wrists seem to be enlarged and there are bumps along his rib cage. CBC and ESR are within normal limits. Parathyroid hormone and alkaline phosphatase are both high. Serum calcium and phosphate are low. The serum Vitamin D 1, 25 is very low.

The most likely diagnosis is

A) Vitamin D deficient rickets
B) Vitamin D dependent rickets Type 1
C) Vitamin D resistant rickets
D) X-linked familial hypophosphatemia
E) Poor compliance with treatment

QUESTIONS: Endocrinology

143) You are evaluating a 2 year old who is walking bow legged, and whose ankles and wrists seem to be enlarged and there are bumps along his rib cage. CBC and ESR are within normal limits. Parathyroid hormone, alkaline phosphatase and Vitamin D 1, 25 are all high. Serum calcium and phosphate are low.

   The most likely diagnosis is:

   A) Vitamin D deficient rickets
   B) Vitamin D dependent rickets Type 1
   C) Vitamin D resistant rickets
   D) X-linked familial hypophosphatemia
   E) Renal disease

144) Each of the following is associated with metabolic syndrome EXCEPT:

   A) Fasting triglycerides greater than 150
   B) High density lipoprotein cholesterol greater than 40
   C) Blood pressure greater than 130/85
   D) Fasting glucose greater than 100
   E) Previously diagnosed type 2 diabetes mellitus

145) A 17-year-old boy is hospitalized because of severe DKA. The patient is on appropriate insulin regimen as prescribed by the endocrinologist. An appropriate diet has been set up by a nutritionist. You review the old chart and note this is his 5th admission for DKA in the past 5 months. Which of the following is the MOST likely cause of the recurrent DKA?

   A) Inappropriate insulin dosing
   B) Dawn effect
   C) Excessive caloric intake
   D) Somogyi effect
   E) Poor compliance

146) Which of the following statements is TRUE regarding diabetes in children?

A) Type 1 diabetes is strictly an autoimmune phenomenon
B) Type 2 diabetes in children is strictly due to insulin resistance
C) Type 2 diabetes is seen exclusively in obese children.
D) The younger the child, the more likely they have Type 2
E) The younger the child, the more likely they have Type 1

147) In the following set of questions, decide if each numbered choice applies to (A) only, (B) only, both (C), or neither (D):

1) "Incidental" diagnosis on routine physical in asymptomatic patient
2) Vaginal monilial infection can be a presenting sign
3) Acanthosis nigricans
4) Presence of autoantibodies
5) Exacerbated by stress/disease
6) Arcaneis testus

(A) Frequently occurs with Type 1 diabetes
(B) Frequently occurs with Type 2 diabetes
(C) Both
(D) Neither

148) The 7-year-old daughter of a woman with Type 1 diabetes has had several unexplained hypoglycemic seizures. Prior to this time the child had no prior medical problems. Lab studies reveal elevated insulin levels during these hypoglycemic episodes. Which of the following would be MOST useful in determining the cause of the hypoglycemic seizures?

A) Serum islet cell antibody titers
B) Serum ketones
C) Plasma C-peptide concentration
D) Plasma glucagon concentration
E) Serum anti-insulin antibody titers

149) In the following set of questions, decide if each numbered choice applies to (A) only, (B) only, both (C), or neither (D):

1) Hyperthyroidism
2) Hypothyroidism
3) Immune system involvement
4) Precancerous lesion

(A) Graves' disease
(B) Hashimoto's disease
(C) Both
(D) Neither

5) Owned a diner on the 70s hit TV show Happy Days
6) Usually asymptomatic at presentation
7) Can be hypothyroid at presentation

GI

150) Which one of the following can be a contributing factor to chronic non-specific diarrhea in the toddler?

A) High-fat diet
B) Reduced fecal bile acids
C) Juices with equal concentrations of fructose and glucose
D) 2% milk
E) Restricted fluid intake

151) Treatment of chronic non-specific diarrhea would include:

A) Reduction of dietary fiber
B) Cholestyramine
C) Increase of daily fluid intake
D) Replacement of grape and orange juice with apple and pear juice
E) Reduction of fat intake by half

152) Match each GI disorder on the left to its corresponding diagnostic test on the right.

   1) Chronic inflammation   (A) D-xylose absorption study
   2) Pernicious anemia   (B) Elevated ESR
   3) Carbohydrate absorption   (C) CBC
   4) Integrity of intestinal lymphatic system   (D) Stool pH

153) An 18-hour-old infant has bilious stained emesis following 3 initial feedings. The prenatal and delivery history are unremarkable. On physical exam, the infant is quiet. The occasional peristaltic waves are noted and the abdomen is not distended. Which of the following findings is MOST likely on further radiologic evaluation of this infant?

   A) GE reflux
   B) Pyloric hypertrophy
   C) A "double bubble" sign
   D) Malrotation
   E) A choledochal duct cyst

154) Which of the following can be seen with "irritable bowel syndrome"?

   A) Persistent vomiting
   B) Recurrent diarrhea
   C) Short stature
   D) The absence of pain
   E) Hematochezia

155) A 3-year-old boy presents to you with a sudden onset of paroxysmal, colicky pain that started 6 hours ago. The pain comes and goes. He is and has otherwise been healthy. On physical examination there is right upper quadrant tenderness, rectal exam is normal, and stools are guaiac negative. You suspect a diagnosis of intussusception. Each of the following is true regarding intussusception EXCEPT:

   A) A guaiac negative stool can be a result of this being an early presentation
   B) After reduction via air contrast enema, 90% of the time there will be no recurrence
   C) You would expect to find a sausage-like mass on the left lower quadrant
   D) It is the most common cause of intestinal obstruction in children of age 3 months to 6 years.
   E) Bilious vomiting can develop

156) Which of the following is associated with ariboflavinosis?

   A) Cheilosis
   B) Xerophthalmia
   C) Aphonia
   D) Glossitis
   E) Oxaluria

157) A 3-year-old boy presents with recurrrent diarrhea. The child had pneumococcal pneumonia at 1 year of age, and meningitis developed at 2 years of age. IV IgG therapy was initiated 6 months ago. Lab studies show that serum IgG, IgA, and IgM concentrations are decreased. CBC and differential are normal. Which of the following is the MOST likely etiology of the recurrent diarrhea?

   A) Lactase deficiency
   B) Rotavirus infection
   C) *Giardia lamblia* infection
   D) *Entamoeba histolytica* infection
   E) Enterovirus infection

158) One could expect to see low serum albumin levels with each of the following conditions EXCEPT:

   A) Kwashiorkor
   B) Ascites
   C) Inflammatory bowel disease
   D) Nephrotic syndrome
   E) Hepatitis A

159) A 17-year-old varsity quarterback in your practice is at your office for a school physical in early September. He is being pursued by several universities to play football.[5] The football team has already been training since August 8th. With the exception of his being noticeably icteric, his physical examination is benign. He is unfazed and says this happens every football season and then it resolves. Additional history, laboratory, and physical findings are MOST likely to reveal

   A) History of alcohol abuse and severe dehydration
   B) Similar past history in the patient as well as his male siblings[6] with elevated unconjugated bilirubin levels and otherwise normal lab findings
   C) Low hematocrit on CBC with the elevated bilirubin due to hemolysis secondary to low grade crush injuries while getting tackled
   D) Evidence of acute hepatitis A due to the high risk of the team drinking from the same bottles of sports drinks
   E) Evidence of undetected chronic hepatitis B

160) Each of the following has been associated with an increased risk for developing hemolytic uremic syndrome after a child is infected with the causative enterohemorrhagic *E. coli* EXCEPT:

   A) Older age
   B) Use of antimotility medication
   C) Use of antibiotics
   D) Elevated WBC
   E) Presence of prolonged diarrhea

161) A 12-year-old boy was recently treated with amoxicillin for 10 days for *Streptococcus* pharyngitis. One week after amoxicillin is discontinued, severe diarrhea develops. The MOST likely cause of this problem is:

   A) Norwalk viral infection
   B) Shigella infection
   C) Toxin-induced colitis
   D) Immune reaction to antibiotics
   E) Ulcerative colitis

---

[5] And enroll in the gluteus maximus–olecranon process comparative analysis major.
[6] Also known as brothers to the lay public, by the way.

162) Each of the following is true regarding Alpha 1 –antitrypsin deficiency *except*:

   A) It is the most common genetic cause of acute liver disease in children
   B) It is the most common genetic cause of chronic liver disease in children
   C) It is the most common genetically caused disorder necessitating liver transplantation in children
   D) Markedly elevated transaminase values are seen in toddlers
   E) It can present as neonatal hepatitis syndrome in children

163) Which of the following would be the most appropriate management of a 3 month old infant who is spitting up after feedings but is otherwise asymptomatic. The weight and height are at the 60th percentile.

   A) Change to hypoallergenic formula
   B) Thicken formula with rice cereal
   C) Put the infant to sleep in the prone position
   D) Reassure the mother
   E) Start omeprazole

164) Which one of the following is typical of acute gastroenteritis secondary to rotavirus?

   A) Bilious vomiting
   B) Occurrence during the summer
   C) Bloody diarrhea
   D) The absence of respiratory symptoms
   E) Non-bilious vomiting

165) Each of the following is a true statement regarding the most recently licensed vaccines for rotavirus *except:*

   A) They are live vaccines
   B) They have been associated with intussusception
   C) All doses are administered between 2 and 6 months of age
   D) The 3rd dose should not be given later than 32 weeks of age
   E) The 1st dose should be given before 12 weeks of age

Pulmonary

166) Bronchiectasis is best diagnosed by:

   A) Serial chest X rays
   B) Arteriography
   C) Pulmonary function testing
   D) CT scan
   E) Radionucleotide study

167) A 6-month-old former 27 week preemie is failing to thrive (FTT). Caloric intake is appropriate. Medications include multivitamins and albuterol. The infant was weaned from oxygen therapy 2 months ago. Vital signs and the physical examination are normal except for the poor weight gain. CXR findings are consistent with bronchopulmonary dysplasia. Which of the following is the next appropriate step?

   A) Measure oxygen SATs while the infant is sleeping
   B) Restart oxygen therapy
   C) Start Pulmicort® twice a day via nebulizer
   D) Measure sweat chloride
   E) Reassure the mother that this is expected with bronchopulmonary dysplasia

QUESTIONS: Pulmonary

168) A 5-year-old boy presents with 5 months of intermittent fever, fatigue, and weight loss accompanied by coughing. He has just completed a course of amoxicillin with minimal improvement. His appetite and PO intake have been poor. He has a past medical history significant for several upper respiratory infections as well as several bouts of otitis media. His immunizations are all up to date.

According to his mother he has had fever for 5 weeks, the mother notes that she too has had a nagging cough for several months. The boy has had no other associated symptoms such as vomiting, diarrhea, urinary problems, or rash.

On physical examination, his temperature is 38.5 C and his vital signs are stable. HEENT exam is normal except for several palpable 1-cm anterior cervical lymph nodes. Examination of the lungs reveals wheezes and crackles on the right. Physical examination is otherwise normal.

Labs: H/H 14/32, WBC 5, 60 P, 30 L, 10 M, MCV 80, platelets 450, ESR 50, CXR-R perihilar infiltrate, with hilar adenopathy. The *most likely* diagnosis is:

A) Leukemia
B) Pneumococcal pneumonia
C) RSV bronchiolitis
D) Cystic fibrosis
E) *Mycobacterium tuberculosis*

169) The most appropriate next step in confirming the above diagnosis would be:

A) Blood culture
B) CT scan
C) PPD placement
D) Bone marrow biopsy
E) Open lung biopsy

170) A 6-week-old is brought to the ER for evaluation of "noisy breathing" and "choking". The mother notes that this has been going on since birth and their pediatrician has done nothing. She wants you to do something right now!

Growth and development are normal. The infant breast-feeds well. On physical examination, intermittent mild intercostal and subcostal retractions and mild inspiratory stridor are present. There are no wheezing, rales or rhonchi. Which of the following is the *most appropriate* next course of action?

A) pH probe study
B) Reassurance
C) Inspiratory and expiratory x-ray studies of the chest
D) Call the pediatrician at home and ask how he can sleep knowing this child is suffering like this.
E) Pulse oximetry

171) You are evaluating a 9-month-old whose mother claims is "always sick". Which of the following would lead you to believe that this infant may actually have a possible immunodeficiency?

A) Ten upper respiratory tract infections during the past 6 months
B) Three episodes of bilateral otitis media
C) Recurrent "pneumonia" with wheezing
D) Two hospitalizations for febrile pneumonia
E) Severe post-tussive emesis

172) You are called to evaluate an infant in the nursery who becomes cyanotic at rest. The cyanosis clears up with vigorous crying. You suspect a diagnosis of choanal atresia. All of the following are true EXCEPT:

A) Definitive diagnosis is made by the failure to pass an NG tube
B) It may be associated with cardiac malformations
C) It may be associated with ear anomalies.
D) Obstruction of both nares can be life threatening in an infant younger than 5 months
E) Initial treatment is with an oropharyngeal airway.

QUESTIONS: Pulmonary

173) A diagnosis of asthma is supported by a decrease in the forced expiratory volume (FEV$_1$) by at least:

A) 2%
B) 5%
C) 15%
D) 35%
E) 50%

174) Each of the following is true regarding inhaled corticosteroids use in the treatment of asthma EXCEPT:

A) They induce the production of beta 2 receptors, enhancing action of beta 2 agonists such as albuterol
B) They reduce the number of mast cells in cells lining the airway
C) They decrease the synthesis of leukocyte protease inhibitor
D) As many as 50% of patients who are well controlled with inhaled corticosteroids can still experience exercise-induced asthma
E) With an inhaler, up to 80% of the inhaled dose is deposited in the oropharynx

175) The mother of a 9-year-old child reports that he has had at least twelve episodes of "pneumonia" in the fall and winter seasons over the past 4 years. Between episodes, she says that he seems to be healthy, although he has frequent episodes of coughing. His height and weight are at the 30% for age. Scattered, low-pitched wheezes are heard in all lung fields on forced expiration. Findings on x-ray study of the chest are normal except for partial right middle lobe atelectasis. Which of the following is the most likely diagnosis?

A) Reactive airway disease
B) Cystic fibrosis
C) Foreign body aspiration
D) Tension pneumothorax
E) Congenital absence of the secretory component of IgA

176) A patient with acute asthma is most likely to have decreased:

A) Peak expiratory flow rate
B) Residual volume
C) Functional residual capacity
D) Total lung capacity
E) Tidal volume

177) Which of the following statements is true regarding the treatment of acute asthma exacerbations in children?

A) Levalbuterol has not been proven to be superior to racemic albuterol as a first line bronchodilator
B) Bacterial infections are implicated much more commonly as triggers than viral infections
C) It is never appropriate to have a patient maintain a supply of systemic steroids
D) Chest physical therapy should be a part of routine care in asthma exacerbations
E) Inhaled mucolytics should be a part of routine care in asthma exacerbations

178) Each of the following statements is true regarding the mechanism of action of pharmacological agents used to treat asthma *except*:

A) Inhaled cromolyn prevents both the early and late airway response to *allergy triggered* asthma
B) Inhaled steroids help inhibit the early but not the late bronchospastic response
C) Severe early bronchospasms respond promptly to short acting bronchodilators
D) Mast cell activation is responsible for the late bronchospastic response to allergen exposure.
E) Inflammation is the underlying abnormality present in patients who have even mild asthma.

179) You are evaluating a 7 year old with general malaise, low grade fever, headache and dry cough. Chest x-ray reveals bilateral patchy infiltrates. The most likely diagnosis would be:

A) Acute smoke inhalation
B) Bordetella pertussis
C) Bodega pertussis
D) Mycoplasma pneumonia
E) RSV pneumonia

Cardiology

180) All of the following are components of tetralogy of Fallot EXCEPT:

A) Overriding aorta
B) Pulmonary stenosis
C) VSD
D) Tricuspid atresia ✗
E) Right ventricular hypertrophy

181) Match each with the lettered choice that best corresponds to the EKG tracing.

(A) — SR

(B) — SVT

(C) — 3rd → 2nd

(D) — 2nd → 3rd

(E) — VT VF

(F) — VF VT

(G) [ECG tracing labeled "WPW"]

(H) [ECG tracing labeled "PVC"]

1) Ventricular Fibrillation (V-Fib)
2) Ventricular Tachycardia (V-Tach)
3) Wolf Parkinson White syndrome (WPW)
4) Sinus arrhythmia
5) 2nd degree AV block
6) 3rd degree AV block
7) Premature ventricular contraction (PVC)
8) Supraventricular tachycardia (SVT)

182) Match the disease on the left with the heart sounds on the right.

1) Aortic stenosis
2) Pulmonary stenosis
3) Coarctation of the aorta
4) ASD
5) VSD
6) PDA
7) Mitral insufficiency
8) Aortic insufficiency

(A) Fixed splitting of S2
(B) Diastolic decrescendo murmur
(C) Continuous murmur often heard best in the intraclavicular area
(D) Systolic ejection click that does not vary with respiration
(E) Presence of an ejection click that varies with respiration
(F) Holosystolic, or nearly so, and is heard best at the apex
(G) A continuous murmur over the back
(H) Diastolic rumble in mid-diastole, heard best along the lower left sternal border

QUESTIONS: Cardiology

183) Each of the following is a cause of cyanotic heart disease in newborns EXCEPT:

   A) d-Transposition of the great arteries
   B) Truncus arteriosis
   C) Aortic insufficiency
   D) Tricuspid atresia
   E) Anomalous (total) pulmonary venous return

184) A 5-year-old child has a grade 2/6, mid-systolic, musical, medium-pitched cardiac murmur heard best along the left lower and midsternal border. Which of the following is the MOST likely diagnosis?

   A) ASD
   B) MVP
   C) Innocent murmur
   D) Pulmonary valve stenosis
   E) VSD

185) A left axis deviation may be seen on EKG with all of the following EXCEPT:

   A) Coarctation of the aorta
   B) AV canal defects
   C) Tricuspid atresia
   D) Double outlet right ventricle
   E) Hypertrophic cardiomyopathy

186) An acyanotic 2-month-old boy is hospitalized because of irritability, poor feeding, and dyspnea of 7 days' duration. HR is 170/min, RR 60/min. Physical examination reveals a harsh holosystolic murmur associated with a precordial systolic thrill at the lower left sternal border; there is a diastolic rumble at the apex.[7] Crackles are heard in both lung bases. The liver is palpable 3 cm below the right costal margin. Which of the following is the MOST likely diagnosis?

A) VSD
B) ASD
C) Complete transposition of the great arteries
D) Anomalous origin of the left coronary artery
E) TOF

187) The gold standard for diagnosing *subacute bacterial endocarditis* would be:

A) An echocardiogram
B) A 24-hour EKG monitoring
C) Cardiac catheterization
D) A positive blood culture
E) Elevated erythrocyte sedimentation rate

---

[7] Are you ready to rumble?

QUESTIONS: Cardiology

188) The Cardiac cath oxygen saturation and pressure gradient demonstrated below is most consistent with:

A) Normal heart
B) Tetralogy of Fallot
C) Truncus arteriosis
D) Total anomalous venous return
E) Transposition of the great vessels

	(SVC) 70%	98% (PV)	
(RA)	2 70%	5 98%	(LA)
(RV)	110/10 80%	110/10 80%	(LV)
Truncus	110/10 80%	110/10 80%	

189) The Cardiac cath oxygen saturation and pressure gradient demonstrated below is most consistent with:

A) Normal heart
B) Tetralogy of Fallot
C) Total anomalous venous return
D) Pulmonary stenosis
E) Aortic stenosis

	(SVC) 70%	95% (PV)	
(RA)	2 85%	3 85%	(LA)
(RV)	22/2 85%	110/50 85%	(LV)
PA	40/18 85%	110/50 85%	A

QUESTIONS: Cardiology

190) Which of the following is true regarding the management of cardiac complications of Kawasaki disease?

A) High dose aspirin is given during the acute phase and then discontinued
B) Cardiac echo is done when Kawasaki is diagnosed to assess for coronary artery aneurysms
C) Cardiac complications include myocarditis and valvulitis
D) Low dose aspirin is given during the acute phase and then discontinued
E) Intravenous gamma globulin is given during the subacute phase

191) You are evaluating a 16 year old varsity football player who is complaining of sharp left sided chest pain which increases with deep breaths. His grandfather died of a myocardial infarction at age 62 and his 57 year old father is being treated for hypertension. Physical examination is unremarkable.

The most appropriate next step in managing this patient is

A) Trial of antacids no restrictions on playing ball
B) Abdominal CT with IV contrast to assess for cholecystitis
C) Trial of ibuprofen and no restrictions
D) EKG and if no ST changes clear for full activity
E) Cardiology referral and restriction of sports and other strenuous exercise

192) Which of the following would be the most appropriate management of a child with a strong family history of hypercholesterolemia?

A) Implement a low fat diet
B) Implement a low cholesterol diet
C) Measure fasting serum triglycerides and cholesterol
D) Order a cardiac echo
E) Start lipid lowering medication

Heme Onc

193) All of the following are vitamin K dependent clotting factors *EXCEPT*:

   A) 2
   B) 7
   C) 8
   D) 9
   E) 10

194) Each of the following is associated with a poor prognosis in acute lymphocytic leukemia *EXCEPT*:

   A) High white blood cell count
   B) Male gender
   C) Pre-B cell
   D) Young age at diagnosis
   E) Slow response to treatment

195) The parents of a child who had unilateral retinoblastoma would like to know the odds of any subsequent children also having the disorder. You correctly tell them:

   A) 5%
   B) 25%
   C) 50%
   D) 75%
   E) 100%

QUESTIONS: Heme One

196) You are giving a talk on sickle cell disease to the residents. You need to discuss management and association of sickle cell disease and *stroke*. Each of the following from your handout is correct *EXCEPT*:

   A) Exchange transfusion can reduce the incidence of stroke
   B) Subtle neuropsychological deficits often result from focal strokes
   C) 6% of children with sickle cell disease develop strokes
   D) CVA's with sickle cell disease is due to both small and large vessel injury
   E) The most accurate diagnostic assessment can be obtained through head CT

197) Patients who are neutropenic are most vulnerable to:

   A) Opportunistic infections
   B) Fungal infections
   C) Respiratory tract flora
   D) Skin and GI flora
   E) Parasitic infections

198) Which of the following would be the most common cause for isolated neutropenia in a generally healthy patient in your practice?

   A) Poor nutrition
   B) Neutered neutropenia
   C) Acute lymphocytic leukemia
   D) Viral syndrome
   E) Cyclic neutropenia

199) Match the type of anemia on the left to the lab profile on the right. :

			RDW	Ferritin	FEP	TIBC
1)	Anemia of chronic illness	(A)	Elevated	Low	Elevated	Elevated
2)	Beta thalassemia	(B)	Low	Normal	Normal	Normal
3)	Iron deficiency	(C)	Normal	Normal or High	Elevated	Elevated
4)	Lead poisoning	(D)	Decreased	Normal	Elevated	Decreased

200) In the following set of questions, decide if each numbered choice applies to (A) only, (B) only, both (C), or neither (D):

1) X-linked recessive
2) Autosomal dominant
3) Heinz bodies
4) Howell-Jolly bodies
5) Aplastic crisis
6) Autosomal recessive

(A) G 6PD deficiency
(B) Hereditary spherocytosis
(C) Both
(D) Neither

201) In the following set of questions, decide if each numbered choice applies to (A) only, (B) only, both (C), or neither (D):

1) Thrombocytopenia
2) Increased PTT
3) Abnormal platelet function
4) Eczema
5) Recent viral illness
6) At risk for developing malignancies

(A) Wiskott Aldrich syndrome
(B) Idiopathic thrombocytopenic purpura
(C) Both
(D) Neither

202) In the following set of questions, decide if each numbered choice applies to (A) only, (B) only, both (C), or neither (D):

1) Joint pain
2) Bone pain
3) Morning stiffness
4) Lymphadenopathy / hepatosplenomegaly
5) Associated with exposure to microwave towers

(A) JRA
(B) Acute leukemia
(C) Both
(D) Neither

203) An otherwise healthy 12-day-old girl presents with bloody stools. She was born at home and has been exclusively breast-fed. A physician has not yet examined her until now. In addition to a rapid heart rate, you note some blue areas of discoloration on the limbs and buttocks. The rest of the physical exam is unremarkable. The MOST likely diagnosis is:

A) Child abuse
B) Henoch Schönlein purpura
C) Anal fissure
D) Hemorrhagic disease of the newborn
E) Von Willebrand disease

204) Each of the following is associated with Fanconi's anemia EXCEPT:

A) Autosomal recessive inheritance pattern
B) Abnormal skin pigmentation
C) Pancytopenia noted during the first year of life
D) Renal abnormalities
E) Skeletal abnormalities

205) A 2-1/2-year-old is noted to have Horner's syndrome on the right side. A chest x-ray is ordered and a mass in the upper portion of the mediastinum is noted. The MOST likely diagnosis would be:

A) Lymphoma
B) Tuberculosis
C) Acute lymphocytic leukemia
D) Neuroblastoma
E) Wilms' tumor

206) Regarding iron deficiency anemia, all of the following are true EXCEPT:

A) Serum ferritin levels are lowered
B) Serum iron binding capacity is reduced
C) Serum iron levels are reduced
D) Mean corpuscle volume (MCV) is reduced
E) Iron supplementation is the treatment of choice

207) The "cycles" of cyclic neutropenia consist of periods where neutrophil counts go from normal to neutropenic values. The period of time of "normal values: neutropenic values" is closest to:

   A) 1 week normal values: 1 week neutropenic
   B) 3 weeks normal values: 1 week neutropenic
   C) 8 weeks normal values: 2 weeks neutropenic
   D) 16 weeks normal values: 8 weeks neutropenic
   E) 22 light years normal values: 2 hours neutropenic

208) Each of the following is associated with the *typical* anemia seen in hemolytic uremic syndrome EXCEPT:

   A) Schistocytes
   B) Burr cells
   C) Helmet cells
   D) Thrombocytopenia
   E) Coombs-positive

209) A 6-month-old African American infant who has been fed only formula appears pale. Another physician has recently prescribed him iron therapy. HCT is 26% and reticulocyte counts of 12%; blood smear shows normocytic RBCs and some poikilocytosis and target cells. To manage this infant MOST appropriately you would:

   A) Continue iron therapy only
   B) Continue the iron therapy and add folic acid supplements
   C) Order hemoglobin electrophoresis
   D) Discontinue the iron therapy and give folic acid supplements
   E) Order examination of the bone marrow

210) Each of the following would be a possible indication for a red blood cell transfusion in a patient with hereditary spherocytosis *except:*

 A) Hematocrit lower than 24
 B) Severe chronic fatigue
 C) Hypersplenism
 D) Growth retardation
 E) Extramedullary hematopiesis

211) Which of the following lab studies would be *most helpful* in differentiating hereditary spherocytosis from ABO incompatibility hemolytic anemia?

 A) Haptoglobin levels
 B) Unconjugated bilirubin levels
 C) Lactic dehydrogenase levels
 D) Presence of spherocytes on peripheral smear
 E) Direct Coombs

212) Which of the following is true regarding the risk of cardiotoxicity in patients receiving treatment with *anthracycline?*

 A) Males and females are at equal risk
 B) Cardiotoxicity does not occur at relatively low doses
 C) Age of diagnosis is not a factor
 D) Screening is done every 5 years regardless of cumulative dose
 E) Screening is done every 1-5 years depending on cumulative dose

213) Secondary malignancies are particularly common following:

 A) Non-Hodgkin's lymphoma
 B) Hodgkin's Lymphoma
 C) Retinoblastoma
 D) Neuroblastoma
 E) Acute lymphocytic leukemia

214) A 4 year old boy of Mediterranean descent recently treated with an unknown antibiotic for a febrile illness presents with acute onset of pallor. He has not traveled outside the US recently. On physical exam you confirm the pallor and note that the boy is icteric. Abdominal exam is benign, and there is no hepatosplenomegaly. The heart rate is 155. WBC is 12.5, hematocrit is 20.

The most likely explanation for the boy's presentation is:

A) Sickle cell disease
B) Hepatitis A.
C) Hereditary spherocytosis
D) Acute lymphoblastic leukemia
E) G6PD deficiency

215) You are evaluating a 2 year old with a painless abdominal mass noted by the mother while dressing her. The child is otherwise completely asymptomatic. Which of the following is the most likely diagnosis?

A) Wilms tumor
B) Neuroblastoma
C) Hepatoblastoma
D) Toxic megacolon
E) Mesenteric adenitis

216) You are evaluating a 2 year old with fever, irritability, and mild periorbital ecchymoses. On physical examination you note a painless abdominal mass. Which of the following is the most likely diagnosis?

A) Wilms tumor
B) Neuroblastoma
C) Retinoblastoma
D) Acute leukemia
E) Child abuse

QUESTIONS: Renal

217) Each of the following would be considered triggers for a blood transfusion in the absence of physiological compensation *except*:

A) Estimated traumatic blood loss of 15%
B) Estimated surgical blood loss of 15%
C) Hematocrit level below 20
D) Hemoglobin level below 10
E) A and B

Renal

218) All of the following causes of glomerulonephritis are accompanied by low serum complement levels *EXCEPT*:

A) Post-strep glomerulonephritis
B) Membranoproliferative glomerulonephritis
C) Systemic lupus nephritis
D) Focal segmental glomerulosclerosis

219) A 16-year-old boy is seeing you for a pre-sports physical. His previous physical exams and laboratory findings have been within normal limits. His father and uncle both have hypertension. His blood pressure, taken with the proper-sized cuff on 3 separate occasions over 3 months, was between 140/90 mm Hg and 145/95 mm Hg. BP in the left leg was 150/100. Urinalysis, CBC, EKG, and renal studies were all within normal limits. Of the following, the MOST likely diagnosis is:

A) Renal vascular disease
B) Post strep glomerulonephritis
C) Pheochromocytoma
D) Essential hypertension
E) Hyperthyroidism

220) Each of the following are associated with prune belly syndrome EXCEPT:

A) Cryptorchidism in males
B) Ovarian dysplasia in females
C) Decreased abdominal musculature
D) Pulmonary hypoplasia
E) Renal dysplasia

221) A 6-year-old child is transferred to your practice because the parents are not happy with the care he has received elsewhere. The child is in the 4th percentile for both height and weight.[8] Lab results show Sodium of 136, Potassium of 3.2, Chloride of 114, and a serum Bicarb of 10. The Urine pH is 6.7. You win the parents over by noting that the MOST likely diagnosis based on these findings is:

A) Polycystic kidney disease
B) Congenital short stature
C) Metabolic organic acidosis
D) Distal tubular acidosis
E) Proximal tubular acidosis

222) A 4-year-old presents with periorbital and pretibial edema. Blood pressure is noted to be 130/85. Lab results include a BUN of 30, creatinine of 1.2, and albumin of 1.6. The MOST likely diagnosis based on these findings would be:

A) Focal segmental glomerulonephritis
B) Minimal change nephrotic syndrome
C) Lupus nephritis
D) Liver failure
E) Henoch-Schönlein purpura

---

[8] And the parents are in the 95%ile for anger.

QUESTIONS: Renal

223) An 8-year-old girl presents with a history of dysuria for 2 to 3 days. She is afebrile. The urinalysis reveals a urine pH of 8.0 with 4-5 RBC and 10-15 WBC.
The MOST likely organism causing the UTI would be:

   A) E. Coli
   B) Proteus
   C) Tuberculosis
   D) Viral
   E) Klebsiella

224) In addition to an infectious etiology, hemolytic uremic syndrome can also be caused by each of the following EXCEPT:

   A) Inborn error of cobalamin metabolism
   B) Autosomal recessive inheritance
   C) Pregnancy
   D) X-linked recessive inheritance pattern
   E) Oral contraceptive use

225) While hematuria is often a benign incidental finding in children, it can sometimes indicate a glomerular lesion. Which of the following is TRUE regarding hematuria and glomerular disease?

   A) Urine is tea-colored and actually contains tea leaves
   B) The absence of dysmorphic RBCs all but rules out glomerular disease
   C) The presence of casts containing RBCs is the most ominous sign
   D) The presence of serrated RBCs in urinary sediment is the most ominous sign.
   E) A 24-hour calcium/creatinine is required to rule out hypercalciuria as the cause of hematuria.

226) Each of the following renal stones can be seen in plain x-ray *EXCEPT:*

   A) Calcium
   B) Oxalate
   C) Struvite
   D) Uric acid
   E) Cystine

227) Which of the following imaging studies offers the highest sensitivity and specificity in identifying renal stones of various composition and size?

A) Renal Ultrasound
B) IVP
C) Helical nonenhanced CT
D) Helical enhanced CT
E) Plain x-ray

228) Each of the following is true regarding cystine renal stones *except:*

A) Recurrent nephrolithiasis is the only clinical manifestation of cystinuria
B) Cystinuria can be associated with calcium oxalate stones
C) Cystinosis is associated with nephrolithiasis
D) Urine alkalization is part of the treatment
E) Increased fluid intake is part of the treatment

229) Routine ultrasound during pregnancy reveals severe oligohydramnios and bilateral hydronephrosis. What is the most likely explanation for these findings?

A) Prune Belly syndrome
B) Esophageal atresia
C) Premature rupture of membranes
D) Posterior urethral valves
E) Both A and D

230) You are caring for an overweight teenager with elevated blood pressure with an appropriately-sized cuff on 3 separate occasions each one month apart by 3 experienced nurses. Which of the following would be the most appropriate initial steps in managing this patient?

A) Lasix
B) Atenolol
C) Repeat the blood pressure in a week
D) Nutrition and exercise consultation
E) Reassurance that hypertension will resolve

Urinary

231) Each of the following can be explained by an etiology other than sexual abuse in a pre-adolescent girl EXCEPT:

A) Malodorous vaginal discharge
B) Anterior hymenal tears
C) Molluscum contagiosum
D) Vaginal chlamydia trachomatis infection
E) Bacterial vaginosis

232) A 3-year-old boy has swelling, erythema, and a firm tender area in the left scrotum. The right testis is palpable and appears normal. Which of the following is the MOST likely diagnosis?

A) Epididymitis
B) Hydrocele
C) Inguinal hernia
D) Torsion of the appendix testes
E) Varicocele

233) A 4-year-old girl was toilet trained approximately one year ago. She has developed diurnal enuresis noted by her daycare director. The physical examination is normal, and there is nothing stressful in the child's life to precipitate this problem. Which of the following is the MOST appropriate next step?

A) Imipramine therapy
B) MRI of the lumbosacral spine
C) DDAVP therapy when sleeping outside the home
D) Urinalysis
E) Evaluation under anesthesia for ectopic uretal orifice

234) You are evaluating a 2 month old boy who has bilateral scrotal swelling which is completely non tender. Both sides transilluminate. The most likely diagnosis is:

   A) Epididymitis
   B) Bilateral inguinal hernia
   C) Variocele
   D) Hydrocele
   E) Torsion of the testicle

235) A 6-year-old girl presents with mild bloody vaginal discharge. The discharge has become has become increasingly malodorous during the past few days. On physical examination, there is no evidence of trauma. Which of the following is the MOST likely cause of the discharge?

   A) Hemolytic *Streptococcal* infection
   B) Candidal vaginitis
   C) Coagulase-positive *Staphylococcal* infection
   D) Chlamydia vaginitis
   E) Foreign body

236) In which of the following can acute scrotal pain and swelling be seen?

   A) Rocky Mountain Spotted Fever
   B) Henpecked Shoreline purpura
   C) Henoch Schönlein Purpura
   D) Intussusception
   E) Mycoplasma pneumonia

Neurology

237) Each of the following is associated with neurofibromatosis type 1 *EXCEPT*:

A) Acoustic neuromas
B) Lisch nodules
C) Neurofibromas
D) Optic gliomas
E) Learning disabilities

238) Each of the following is true with regards to febrile seizures *EXCEPT*:

A) Neuroimaging is rarely indicated
B) The risk for developing epilepsy in a child who has experienced a complex febrile seizure is slightly higher than that of the general population
C) The risk of developing epilepsy is proportionate to the number of febrile seizures the child has experienced
D) Meningitis must be ruled out clinically in all cases
E) Serum electrolytes, glucose and calcium need not be ordered routinely

239) A 9 year old is being seen in your office for a history of "staring spells" along with weird clicking sounds that some times lead to generalized seizures. After the episodes he is drowsy and out of it. The spells last a minute or two and 2 EEGs have been normal. A head CT, CBC and serum electrolytes are all unremarkable.

Your physical exam is unremarkable. There is no family history of seizures. This history is *most* consistent with a diagnosis of:

A) Absence seizures
B) Tourette syndrome
C) Rolandic seizures
D) Conversion disorder
E) Partial complex seizures

240) A 3 month old in your practice hasn't been eating well and is lethargic. Head circumference is in the 96th percentile and weight is in the 6th percentile, giving him the appearance of a Klingon on *Star Trek the Next generation*. Chest x- ray reveals significant cardiomegaly. A head CT with contrast reveals large ventricles with the 3rd ventricle compressed by a mass. This is confirmed by the radiologist who dictates this while taking a swig from her 5th triple mocha latte of the morning. You simultaneously shout out the *CORRECT* diagnosis:

A) Dandy Walker cyst
B) Epidural hematoma
C) VSD
D) Vein of Galen malformation
E) Subdural hematoma

241) Match each number to its associated seizure on the right.

1) 3 per second spike and wave EEG pattern
2) Hypsarrhythmia pattern on EEG
3) Lip smacking
4) Occur at night

(A) Complex partial seizures
(B) Absence seizures
(C) Infantile spasms
(D) Rolandic seizures

242) Match each number to its corresponding dyskinesia on the right:

1) Smooth movements of the extremities
2) Rapid rhythmic movements
3) Twisting, assuming postures
4) Brief muscle jerking movements
5) Brief movements of the face and shoulder
6) Excessive ants-in-the-pants-like movements

(A) Chorea
(B) Dystonia
(C) Hyperactivity
(D) Myoclonus
(E) Tics
(F) Tremor

QUESTIONS: Neurology

243) A 15-year-old girl presents with a severe headache that began suddenly earlier today. The headache is severe and constant over the left side of her head. In addition, she is complaining about right-sided weakness, especially on the upper extremity. She has had no significant past history and takes no medication routinely. There is no family history of neurologic disease.

She is afebrile, and BP is 115/80 mm Hg. She is having difficulty with neck flexion, with positive Kernig and Brudzinski signs. She is lethargic and responds slowly to both verbal and visual stimuli. A right hemiparesis coupled with hyperreflexia is noted. Eye examination shows no papilledema, no evidence of a visual field deficit, and no sensory abnormalities. Head CT shows a hematoma in the posterolateral portion of the left frontal lobe.
The MOST likely diagnosis is:

A) Cerebral aneurysm
B) Spinal meningitis
C) Subdural hematoma
D) Acute Encephalitis
E) Intracranial hemorrhage due to AV malformation

244) A 9-year-old girl presents with progressive generalized weakness and increasing bilateral ptosis over the past 2-3 months.

The parents note that the weakness gets worse over the course of the day. Fatigue sets in even with minimal physical activity. By evening her voice is weak and she has difficulty swallowing. Vision is normal except for occasional diplopia. The patient has had no fever, pain, rash, or joint swelling. She is receiving no medications.

Her birth history, prenatal history, and developmental history are all normal. Family history is negative for any neuromuscular disease.

On physical examination, you note mild bilateral ptosis, weakness of the left abducens nerve manifested by the inability to move the eye laterally, along with a diminished gag reflex. There is a nasal tone to her voice, suggesting laryngeal muscle weakness. She also has mild weakness of the extremities and notable muscle fatigue with repetitive tasks. CBC and differential are normal. The *most likely* diagnosis is:

A) Myasthenia gravis
B) Guillain-Barré syndrome
C) Multiple sclerosis
D) Botulism poisoning
E) Polio

245) **This illness is due to:**

   A) A virus
   B) Antibodies
   C) Myelin deterioration
   D) Inhibition of neurotransmitter release
   E) Toxin

246) **The MOST appropriate management would be:**

   A) Conservative management
   B) Antibiotic therapy
   C) Antiviral agents
   D) Antitoxin
   E) Cholinesterase inhibitors

247) **A 6-month-old boy has been exhibiting abnormal movements and has been brought to you by the anxious parents. On physical examination, you note sudden flexion of the trunk as well as the neck and limbs. This is followed by gradual relaxation. EEG shows a hypsarrhythmic pattern. Of the following, the *most appropriate* treatment for this condition would be:**

   A) Phenytoin
   B) Adrenocorticotropic hormone (ACTH)
   C) Carbamazepine
   D) Phenobarbital
   E) Valproate

248) **A 15-year-old boy is brought to the ED after a generalized seizure that lasted 20 minutes. Physical examination shows a diminished sensorium and deviation of both eyes to the left. The BEST explanation for these findings is:**

   A) Postictal state
   B) New York state of mind
   C) Persistent seizure activity
   D) Intranuclear ophthalmoplegia
   E) Right-sided brain stem infarct

249) A 10 year old girl presents with a history of a left sided headache along with paresthesias and weakness of the right arm and leg. Preceding the headache she saw specks of light floating in her visual field. She has no difficulty speaking and the headache is still present during the exam. The mother notes that several members of her family suffer from severe migraine headaches.

The most likely diagnosis is

A) Confusional migraine
B) Basilar type migraine
C) Craniopharyngioma
D) Post viral labyrinthitis
E) Familial hemiplegic migraine

250) The parents of a 7 year old boy are concerned over a school report that describes several episodes where he turns his head followed by his eyes blinking. During the episodes he is fully aware of his surroundings and alert. The parents have also noticed similar episodes at home which have occurred on a daily basis for over a year.

In addition he has been noted to sniff during class which has continued despite being asked to stop repeatedly.

The most likely diagnosis would be:

A) Tic disorder
B) Tourette syndrome
C) Absence seizures
D) Attention deficit hyperactivity disorder
E) Allergic rhinitis

251) Which one of the following is true regarding teenagers with a history of epilepsy?

A) Bathing in a tub is prohibited
B) Before withdrawing from medications, a normal EEG must be obtained
C) Juvenile myoclonic epilepsy requires lifetime treatment
D) Driving is prohibited for lifetime
E) Driving is acceptable if seizure free for at least 24 months while on anticonvulsants

252) You are caring for a toddler who has just experienced his first febrile seizure. Which of the following would increase his risk of developing epilepsy?

   A) First febrile seizure before age 1
   B) Low degree of fever at the onset of the seizure
   C) Family history of febrile seizures
   D) Family history of epilepsy
   E) Male gender

Musculoskeletal

253) All of the following are true of, or associated with, Duchenne's muscular dystrophy *EXCEPT*:

   A) Pseudohypertrophy of the calves
   B) X-linked recessive inheritance
   C) Gowers sign
   D) Always inherited from the mother
   E) Proximal muscle weakness

254) A 16 year old girl is referred to your office from her private high school because of "severe scoliosis" noted on routine screening. A 19-degree angle of thoracis scoliosis is noted.

   Your note to the school nurse, confirms that you will:

   A) Suggest physical therapy and twice weekly Rolfing massage at spa beach resort
   B) Confirm the findings with MRI and refer to neurology for follow-up
   C) Repeat films in 6 months
   D) Repeat films in 2 years
   E) Prescribe bracing and followup every 2 months

255) An 8 year old has had a decreased level of energy with a low-grade fever over the past 14 days. On physical exam you note that she is able to walk but is unable to run up flight of stairs and prefers to just lie down on the couch "like her father" according to the mother's description. You also note that her eyelids and cheeks have a reddish color to them. This disorder would *BEST* be treated with:

A) Antitoxin
B) Supportive measures
C) Steroids
D) Immunophoresis
E) IV gamma globulins

256) An 11-year-old soccer player sustained a Salter-Harris I fracture of his left ankle during a game yesterday. He injured the same ankle during a basketball game 9 months earlier. Which of the following is the *most likely* explanation for this child's current injury?

A) Incomplete healing of the old injury
B) Second unrelated injury
C) Osteolytic fracture
D) Osteochondritis dissecans
E) Conversion disorder

257) Each of the following is a common findings with temporomandibular joint (TMJ) dysfunction **EXCEPT:**

A) Tinnitus
B) Preauricular pain
C) Otalgia
D) Swelling of the TMJ
E) Decreased motion of the jaw

258) Each of the following is a risk factor for the development of slipped capital femoral epiphysis (SCFE) EXCEPT:

A) Hypothyroidism
B) Elevated estrogen levels
C) Elevated testosterone levels
D) Male gender
E) African-American race

259) The *most common* benign bone tumor in children is:

A) Osgood-Schlatter's disease
B) Osteogenic sarcoma
C) Osteoid osteoma
D) Ewing's sarcoma
E) Osteochondroma

260) In counseling the parents of a child with achondroplasia, which of the following statements would be most appropriate?

A) The disorder is inherited as an autosomal recessive trait
B) Normal mental development is likely
C) Ventricular shunting will most likely be necessary
D) Bladder and bowel control is rarely affected
E) Chromosome analysis is indicated

QUESTIONS: Musculoskeletal

261) You are evaluating a 3 year old boy who wakes up several times a week complaining of bilateral pain in his shins. He has not had a recent viral illness. He is afebrile and experiences no pain during the day. There is no joint swelling, tenderness, discoloration, or limited range of motion.

   The most likely diagnosis is

   A) Osteoid osteoma
   B) Legg Calve Perthes
   C) Toxic synovitis
   D) Slipped capital femoral epiphysis
   E) Growing pains

262) Which of the following is true regarding Legg Calve Perthes disease?

   A) X-rays are extremely sensitive in detecting early disease
   B) Onset after puberty carries a better prognosis
   C) It frequently occurs in boys between ages 4-10
   D) Boys tend to have a higher prevalence of bilateral disease
   E) Bilateral disease is associated with more severe disease and a worse prognosis

263) You are evaluating a limping 13 year old obese linebacker boy for his school team. He reports left knee pain over 2 weeks which increased when he came down wrong on his ankle while playing basketball. While supine, his leg is externally rotated and slightly flexed. You have a hard time internally rotating his hip secondary to pain. The most likely diagnosis is:

   A) Legg Calve Perthes
   B) Osgood Schlatter
   C) Slipped capital femoral epiphysis
   D) Septic arthritis
   E) Deep tissue hemangioma

264) Idiopathic scoliosis in adolescents is:

A) Inherited in an autosomal recessive pattern
B) X-linked dominant pattern
C) X-linked recessive pattern
D) Behavioral secondary to poor posture
E) Due to numerous factors

265) You are asked to diagnose a child suspected of having Duchenne muscular dystrophy. You will conduct the listed diagnostic studies in which order?

A) Muscle biopsy, genetic analysis, creatinine kinase levels
B) Muscle biopsy, creatinine kinase levels, genetic analysis
C) Genetic analysis, creatinine kinase levels, muscle biopsy
D) Creatinine kinase levels, genetic analysis, muscle biopsy
E) Creatinine kinase levels, muscle biopsy, genetic analysis

266) You are evaluating an infant with internally rotated feet. You correctly diagnose idiopathic talipes equinovarus (club foot). The most likely cause is:

A) Multifactorial
B) Fetal positioning
C) Normal finding
D) X-linked recessive inheritance
E) Autosomal recessive inheritance

267) Conservative management of congenital talipes equinovarus or club foot is:

A) A roundtrip ticket to club foot in the Caribbean
B) Physical therapy
C) Binding via tape
D) Casting and splinting
E) Muscle relaxants for 3 months

Dermatology

268) In the following set of questions, for each numbered word or phrase, choose the lettered heading that is MOST CLOSELY ASSOCIATED with it. Lettered headings may be selected once, more than once, or not at all.

1) Inflammation and black dots
2) Complete areas of smooth hair loss
3) Incomplete patches of hair loss with hair shafts of varying lengths
4) Eyebrows are involved
5) Pediatrician preparing for the Boards

(A) Alopecia neurotica
(B) Alopecia totalis
(C) Trichotillomania
(D) Tinea capitis
(E) Alopecia areata

269) A 15-year-old presents with inflammation and severe tenderness and itching of the lateral toe webs and soles of both feet. There is also a foul odor that often "clears the room". There are fissures noted between the toes as well. His 16-year-old brother has similar symptoms. Which of the following is the most likely diagnosis?

A) Scabies
B) Atopic dermatitis
C) Chemical irritation
D) Hyperhidrosis
E) Tinea pedis

270) The rash MOST associated with fifth disease is:

A) Erythema multiforme
B) Erythema marginatum
C) Erythema nodosum
D) Erythema migrans
E) Erythema infectiosum

271) Which one of the following is associated with bacterial sepsis due to *Neisseria meningitidis* secondary to acquired protein C deficiency?

A) Erythema multiforme
B) Erythema migrans
C) Erythema marginatum
D) Gianotti-Crosti syndrome
E) Purpura fulminans

272) A 9-year-old child presents with tender erythematous nodules on the lower extremities concentrated on the pretibial area. The nodules are very tender. The MOST likely cause of this rash is:

A) Playing goalie without goalie pads
B) Tuberculosis
C) Inflammatory bowel disease
D) Coccidioidomycosis
E) Group A *Strep*

273) A 3-month-old infant presents with a severe rash concentrated on the face and scalp. The rash is yellow in color and scaly, with patches that are ulcerated and crusting. Some petechiae and purpura are noted as well. The BEST step in managing this problem would be:

A) Reassurance
B) Zinc supplements
C) Hydrocortisone cream and nystatin ointment
D) Moisturizing lotions and soap
E) Skin biopsy

274) You are called by the local nurse practitioner who is baffled by a rash in a 4-year-old patient. The nurse describes the rash as flat, non-pruritic papules on the face and extremities, and also notes some lesions on the buttocks, but not the trunk. You, of course, tell her that the diagnosis is:

A) Psoriasis
B) Atopic dermatitis
C) Erythema multiforme
D) Erythema erythema
E) Gianotti-Crosti syndrome

275) Treatment of tinea capitis with oral griseofulvin should include:

A) Lipid-containing foods at the time the medication is given
B) Baseline complete blood count and liver function tests
C) A trial of antifungal shampoo and other agents before using any oral agent
D) Fat-free foods at the time of administration
E) Topical steroids

276) A 15-year-old boy has a large number of comedones on his face, but no papules or pustules. Of the following, the treatment of choice for this boy is:

A) A regimen of face scrubbing with soap and a washcloth
B) The application of mentholated cream as a cleanser
C) The application of retinoic acid cream to his face
D) Oral administration of high doses of vitamin A
E) Oral administration of tetracycline

Rheumatology

277) All of the following are appropriate for preventing recurrences of rheumatic fever *EXCEPT*:

   A) Benzathine penicillin G IM
   B) Penicillin V PO
   C) Cefaclor PO
   D) Erythromycin PO
   E) Sulfadiazine

278) A child who is new to your practice comes in for his first appointment. He has been diagnosed in the past with acute rheumatic fever. The mom brings in an 8-foot high pile of downloaded printouts, miraculously, the forklift and pallets leave only 2 or 3 scratches in your paneling so you tip the forklift operator handsomely.

   She wants know the primary *long-term* concerns she should have about her son. You tell her:

   A) Permanent joint damage caused by the migratory polyarthritis
   B) The effects of mitral valve insufficiency
   C) Aortic insufficiency leading to heart failure
   D) Chronic pain secondary to the subcutaneous nodules
   E) The marginal lifestyle of those exhibiting erythema marginatum

279) The earliest sign of Kawasaki disease is:

   A) Strawberry daiquiri tongue
   B) An obsessive desire to drive a motorcycle
   C) High persistent fever
   D) Non-purulent conjunctivitis
   E) Peeling skin on hands and feet

QUESTIONS: Rheumatology

280) Each of the following is among the major Jones criteria for diagnosing rheumatic fever with the *EXCEPTION* of:

   A) Migratory arthritis
   B) Carditis
   C) Erythema marginatum
   D) Erythema infectiosum
   E) Subcutaneous nodules

281) Match each number (synovial fluid description) to its diagnosis on the right

   1) Clear, WBC < 200
   2) Clear, WBC < 2000, increased viscosity
   3) Cloudy, 5000 WBC, decreased viscosity
   4) Cloudy, 20,000 WBC, decreased viscosity
   5) Yellow, 200,000 decreased viscosity
   6) Yellow, bouquet with a kick and a slight after-taste, 10,000 + epithelial cells

   (A) Kendall Jackson Chardonnay
   (B) JRA
   (C) Normal joint fluid aspirate
   (D) Rheumatic fever
   (E) Septic arthritis
   (F) Trauma

282) Match the numbered condition on the left with the lettered indicator or causative factor on the right.

   1) Mixed connective tissue disease
   2) Antiphospholipid syndrome
   3) Wegener's granulomatosis
   4) Schönlein-Henoch purpura
   5) Systemic lupus erythematosus

   (A) False-positive VDRL
   (B) Systemic vasculitis
   (C) IgA nephropathy
   (D) Antibodies to Smith antigen (anti-SM)
   (E) High titers of antibodies to an RNase-sensitive component of extractable nuclear antigen

283) The vast majority of children with hypermobility syndrome[9] will:

A) Need a cardiac evaluation to evaluate for mitral prolapse, aneurysms, and aortic dissection common with connective tissue disorders
B) Need a complete ophthalmological workup to rule out lens dislocation and iritis
C) Never come to your attention at all
D) Require extensive genetic and metabolic workup
E) Be well known to the lobby security guard[10] and your office staff because of their "cocktail party personality" and playful demeanor

284) Each of the following is a hematological manifestation of systemic lupus erythematosus *except*:

A) Anemia of chronic illness
B) Hemolytic anemia
C) Thrombocytopenia
D) Leukocytosis
E) Leukopenia

285) Which one of the following manifestations of neonatal lupus erythematosus is irreversible?

A) Thrombocytopenia
B) Congenital heart block
C) Cutaneous lupus lesions
D) Hepatitis
E) Hepatomegaly

286) Each of the following medications is used to treat various manifestations of lupus *except:*

A) Non steroidal anti inflammatory medications
B) Glucocorticosteroid
C) Insulin
D) Sunscreen
E) Cyclophosphamide

---

[9] Double-jointed, as it is commonly known on playgrounds.
[10] The one with the pencil-thin mustache and odd-smelling cologne.

Ophthalmology

287) You are evaluating a 5-year-old boy who presents with bilateral mucopurulent eye discharge and is afebrile. On examination you note an injected bulging right tympanic membrane and you diagnose conjunctivitis-otitis media syndrome. His immunizations are up to date. Which of the following organisms is the most likely cause?

   A) *Candida albicans*
   B) Adenovirus
   C) *Chlamydia trachomatis*
   D) *H. Influenzae*
   E) *Staphylococcus aureus*

288) A 3-year-old boy presents with excessive tearing. There is no known history of trauma. In addition, he has had a runny nose, mild sore throat and shoddy cervical lymphadenopathy noted on physical examination. The most appropriate management at this time would be:

   A) Referral to ophthalmologist
   B) Symptomatic supportive measures
   C) Fluorescein stain to assess for corneal abrasion
   D) Oral amoxicillin/clavulanate
   E) Moxifloxacin eyedrops

289) You are called into the triage area to evaluate a patient who notes that his left eye began bothering him less than an hour ago. On examination you note purulent discharge and pseudomembrane formation. There is also significant preauricular lymphadenopathy. What is the most likely cause of this presentation?

   A) Vernal conjunctivitis
   B) Syphilitic conjunctivitis
   C) Ligneous conjunctivitis
   D) Neisseria meningitidis
   E) Giant papillary conjunctivitis

290) A 5 year old boy presents during spring break with left sided swelling of his upper eyelid. He is afebrile and denies any trauma. There is a moderate amount of edema, swelling, erythema and vesiculation of the skin. The eyelid is pruritic, not warm to touch, and non tender. He can partially open the eye revealing a non-injected conjunctiva with no discharge.

The most likely diagnosis to explain swelling would be:

A) Periorbital cellulitis
B) Orbital cellulitis
C) Corneal abrasion
D) Mucopurulent conjunctivitis
E) Contact dermatitis

291) The most appropriate treatment for this 5 year old patient would be:

A) Watchful observation
B) Oral antibiotics
C) IV antibiotics
D) Moxifloxacin eyedrops
E) Cool compresses and topical mild steroid cream

292) A 5 year old presents with swelling, redness, warmth, and tenderness of his left eyelid. He may have been bitten by a mosquito a couple of days ago. He has a low grade fever but is otherwise asymptomatic. His extraocular movements are intact; the conjunctiva is not injected and has no discharge. Visual acuity is grossly intact. The most likely diagnosis would be:

A) Periorbital cellulitis
B) Orbital cellulitis
C) Corneal abrasion
D) Mucopurulent conjunctivitis
E) Insect Bite/ Allergic reaction

293) The most appropriate treatment for this patient would be:

A) Oral antibiotics
B) IV antibiotics
C) Overnight eye patch and follow-up the next day
D) Moxifloxacin eyedrops for 5 days
E) Benadryl and cold compresses

ENT

294) Over-the-counter expectorants generally:

A) Have a substantial antitussive *and* decongestive effect
B) Clinically decrease the viscosity of mucous secretions
C) Have the same effect as compressed powdered candy
D) Increase the volume of secretions but do not affect the viscosity
E) Have an antitussive effect and should be recommended for bedtime use only

295) Tonsils usually reach their maximum size in children at what age?

A) 1 to 1-1/2 years
B) 2 to 3 years
C) 5 to 7 years
D) 10 to 12 years
E) 16 to 18 years

296) An 18-month-old boy has a bark-like cough and inspiratory stridor. An x-ray study of the soft tissue of the neck shows subglottic narrowing. Based on these clinical and radiological findings, the MOST likely diagnosis is:

A) Bacterial tracheitis
B) Epiglottitis
C) Viral croup
D) Subglottic hemangioma
E) Foreign body aspiration

297) A 2-year-old boy presents with a history of purulent nasal discharge from the left nostril for one week. Physical examination reveals copious foul-smelling discharge with some edema of the nares. The MOST likely diagnosis is:

A) Unilateral choanal atresia
B) Bacterial sinusitis
C) Allergic rhinitis
D) Juvenile angiofibroma
E) Foreign body

298) A 5-year-old girl presents with pain behind her ear for 2 days. On physical examination, she has a temperature of 39.8C, and you note swelling over the postauricular area with outward and downward displacement of the pinna. Which of the following is the MOST likely diagnosis?

A) Mastoiditis
B) Parotiditis
C) Mumps
D) Otitis media with effusion
E) Cholesteatoma

299) An 8-year-old develops acute onset of bilateral hearing loss confirmed as sensorineural. The MOST likely cause of this problem would be:

A) Drug toxicity
B) Viral illness
C) Previously undetected bilateral acoustic neuromas
D) Foreign body
E) Autoimmune disease

300) Tympanometry would be MOST useful when used to:

A) Diagnose otitis media
B) Diagnose otitis externa
C) Identify source of middle ear effusion
D) Identify conductive hearing loss
E) Diagnose impaired mobility of the tympanic membrane

301) Which of the following would be the most appropriate antibiotic to use to treat a dental abscess in a 5 year old?

A) Ciprofloxacin
B) Clindamycin
C) Penicillin
D) Augmentin
E) Ceclor

302) The most appropriate intervention in a 15 month old who is bottle and breast fed and has developed dental caries would be to:

A) Discontinue nocturnal breast feeding
B) Continue breastfeeding but have mom take fluoride supplementation
C) Discontinue bottle feeding at night
D) A and C
E) Start vitamins with fluoride

303) Which of the following is the most common complication of otitis media?

   A) Hearing loss
   B) Mastoiditis
   C) Meningitis
   D) Sinusitis
   E) Intracranial abscess

304) A 12 year old presents with several months of nasal congestion, along with a persistent cough at night that keeps him up. He also has been experiencing malaise, poor appetite, intermittent fever and headache. The most likely diagnosis would be:

   A) Allergic rhinitis
   B) Aseptic meningitis
   C) Encephalopathy
   D) Chronic sinusitis
   E) Acute sinusitis

305) A child presents with bilateral ear pain, a low grade fever, erythematous TM, with good movement with insufflation, distinct landmarks and a peaked curve on tympanometry would suggest which diagnosis and treatment?

   A) Otitis media / amoxicillin
   B) Otitis media/ amoxicillin – clavulanic acid
   C) Otitis externa/ cortisone based ear drops
   D) Myringitis/ ibuprofen
   E) Viral infection/ no treatment

306) Appropriate antibiotic treatment of conjunctivitis and otitis media would be:

   A) Amoxicillin
   B) Amoxicillin/ clavulanic acid
   C) Gentamicin eyedrops and amoxicillin
   D) Antibiotic eardrops and eyedrops
   E) Supportive care only

QUESTIONS: Adolescent Medicine and Gynecology

307) You are evaluating a 17 year old female for a sore throat of 5 days duration. Rapid strep and throat culture for Group a beta hemolytic strep was negative. She is sexually active She was treated for a cervical chlamydia infection last month. On physical examination you note red patches of the pharynx, with no exudate and no petechiae.

The most appropriate test to establish a diagnosis would be:

A) Chlamydia throat culture
B) Chlamydia and gonorrhea nucleic acid amplification screening
C) Gonorrhea throat culture
D) Serum monospot
E) No treatment or diagnosing testing

Adolescent Medicine and Gynecology

308) You are asked to help manage a teenage female who is being admitted for anorexia nervosa who is currently 35% below ideal body weight. With regard to rapid refeeding, which of the following should you be MOST concerned about?

A) Hypokalemia
B) Hyperkalemia
C) Hyperphosphatemia
D) Hypophosphatemia
E) Hyponatremia

309) Which of one the following factors is MOST associated with early initiation of sexual activity in teenagers?

A) Higher socioeconomic status
B) Access to condoms in school based clinic
C) Sexual abuse
D) Late onset of puberty
E) Firm parental discipline at home

310) **Which of the following should be kept in mind when counseling teenagers regarding high risk behavior?**

   A) Adolescents have a high capacity for abstract thinking
   B) Long term impacts of poor health habits are a strong deterrent to adolescents
   C) Linking cause and effect regarding health habits over several visits will gradually impact behavior
   D) Reinforcing the impact the behavior will have on their appearance and physical performance compared with their peers should be emphasized
   E) Having them sign a contract with their parents that they will refrain from high risk behavior will ensure the teenager will abstain from the behavior

311) **Which of the following is true regarding sexual orientation in teenagers?**

   A) Transient homosexual experimentation is uncommon
   B) Adolescents who are emotionally attracted to members of the same gender usually engage in sexual activity
   C) Adolescents struggling with issues of sexual identity should be discouraged from doing so
   D) Approximately 30% of gay youths have attempted suicide at least once
   E) Depression and suicide ideation are rare among homosexual teenagers

312) **Which of the following is true regarding scoliosis in teenagers?**

   A) Scoliosis is by definition curvature of the spine greater than 15 degrees
   B) Adolescent idiopathic scoliosis is defined as scoliosis whose onset is seen in children older than 15
   C) Idiopathic scoliosis is more common in boys than girls
   D) Mild – moderate pulmonary compromise can be seen in spine curvature greater than 60 degrees
   E) Adolescent scoliosis is mostly associated with X-linked disorders

QUESTIONS: Adolescent Medicine and Gynecology

313) Each of the following is a true statement regarding sexually transmitted diseases EXCEPT:

A) Chlamydia trachomatis and Neisseria gonorrhea are often asymptomatic in males
B) Chlamydia trachomatis and Neisseria gonorrhea are often asymptomatic in females
C) 50% of sexually active adolescents become infected with sexually transmitted diseases each year
D) Chronic pelvic pain can be a manifestation of PID
E) It is now possible to diagnose Chlamydia trachomatis and Neisseria gonorrhea using urine-based diagnostic testing

314) Each of the following is a significant consideration in the differential diagnosis of anovulatory uterine bleeding in an adolescent female EXCEPT:

A) Hyperthyroidism
B) Hypothyroidism
C) Cystic fibrosis
D) Hyperprolactinemia
E) Disordered eating

315) You are evaluating a 16 year old female who is new to your practice. She has been experiencing heavy, painless monthly bleeding since the onset of menses. There is a significant family history for heavy menstrual bleeding in the family including the patient's mother. She is physically active, height and weight are both in the 60th percentile and her SMR is 5. The most likely explanation for the heavy menstrual bleeding would be:

A) Factor VIII deficiency
B) Factor IX deficiency
C) Von Willebrand disease
D) Polycystic ovary syndrome
E) Crohn's disease

Sports Medicine

316) Which of the following would be consistent with androstenedione use in a teenage athlete?

   A) Lowered estradiol levels
   B) Elevated testosterone levels
   C) Elevated high-density lipoproteins
   D) Decreased high density proteins
   E) Decreased serum lipid levels

317) Please match the clinical description on the right with the likely drug / supplement / medication on the left

   1) Creatinine supplement
   2) Anabolic Androgenic steroids
   3) Guarana extract

   A) Increased alertness, headaches and anxiety
   B) Fatigue, abdominal pain, water retention and weight gain
   C) Muscle hypertrophy and increased number of muscle fibers
   D) Decreased urine luteinizing hormone

318) All of the following are effective deterrents to the inappropriate use of performance enhancing drugs in teenagers except:

   A) Maintaining an open dialogue
   B) Testing them to show them their low sperm count due to anabolic androgenic steroids
   C) Drug testing
   D) Encouraging proper nutrition
   E) Encouraging and providing guidance for proper training

Substance Abuse

319) The most widely used drug among teenagers is:

A) PCP
B) Ecstasy
C) Alcohol
D) Marijuana
E) Love

320) You are evaluating a 16 year old boy in the ER who returned home late from a party. He is very anxious, restless and animated. He is complaining of abdominal cramping. On physical examination you note mydriasis, tachycardia, mild hypertension and increased deep tendon reflexes.

Which of the following would explain the patient's behavior?

A) Undiagnosed bipolar disease
B) Amphetamine abuse
C) PCP abuse
D) Alcohol toxicity
E) Cannabis abuse

321) You are evaluating a 15 year old boy who reportedly had been smoking marijuana possibly laced with PCP. On physical exam he is disoriented and stares blankly. His muscles are rigid. He is slightly tachycardic with elevated blood pressure. The most appropriate next step in managing this patient would be:

A) Place patient in a windowless secure room
B) Provide rectal Valium
C) Measure serum myoglobin
D) Administer naloxone intramuscularly
E) Acidify his urine

322) Which of the following is true regarding drug use in the United States?

A) Drug use among high school students was at its highest in the 1980s
B) Cigarette smoking among 8th-12 graders has increased over the past decade
C) The use of performance enhancing drugs decreases the likelihood of use of other illicit drugs
D) Homosexual adolescents have rates of substance abuse that are significantly higher than heterosexual peers
E) Inhalant abuse is more prevalent among 12th graders than 8th graders

323) You are asked to medically clear a teenage boy for a psychiatric evaluation. Over the past few weeks he has had violent outbursts and has exhibited hypomania.

His blood pressure is 125/85 and he is built like a football player. You note on physical exam the presence of acne, primarily pustular –papular as well as bilateral gynecomastia. His voice is higher pitched than would be expected for his Tanner stage.

The abuse of which of the following substances is the likely explanation?

A) The refrigerator
B) Marijuana
C) Methylphenidate
D) Anabolic steroids
E) Growth hormone

Disorders of Cognition, Language & Learning

324) With regards to learning disabilities in children, all of the following are true EXCEPT:

A) The most common forms of learning disabilities are reading disorders and dyslexia.
B) Grade retention is a favored approach in learning disabilities.
C) Diagnosis is based on history and neuro-psychometric testing.
D) A learning disability can coexist with an above average IQ.
E) Most learning disabilities resolve by early adulthood.

325) During a routine physical you note that the child you are examining can walk upstairs with one hand held and turn the pages of your textbook 3 pages at a time. The parents tell you that he can speak 10 words and can identify 1 body part. The child's age is closest to:

A) 16 months
B) 18 months
C) 24 months
D) 30 months
E) 36 months

326) Which of the following is true regarding intellectual disability in children?

A) 25% of children with severe intellectual disability have associated behavioral problems
B) Seizures are twice as common in children who have intellectual disability than the general population
C) Approximately 25% of patients with cerebral palsy have comorbid intellectual disability of some degree
D) The correct term for children less than 6 years old suspected of having intellectual disability is *global developmental delay*
E) The prevalence of sleep disorders is proportional to intelligence

327) **Which of the following is true regarding eligibility for Early Intervention Programs (EIP)?**

   A) Infants diagnosed with a syndrome known to be associated with intellectual disability become eligible when developmental delays are identified

   B) Infants diagnosed with a syndrome known to be associated with intellectual disability become eligible at age 3

   C) Infants diagnosed with a syndrome known to be associated with intellectual disability become eligible at birth

   D) Children with developmental concerns should be referred to EIP when they turn 3

   E) Children with developmental concerns should be referred to EIP just prior to entering school

328) **Which of the following statements is true regarding dyslexia ?**

   A) If discovered early, it can be prevented
   B) Dyslexia, by definition, is idiopathic
   C) Vision therapy is the most effective method to overcome dyslexia
   D) Reading aloud to the child is the best method to promote reading skills
   E) Environmental factors do not impact dyslexia

329) **Each of the following activities would be appropriately encouraged in children with autism spectrum disorder *except*:**

   A) Lacrosse
   B) Karate
   C) Swimming
   D) Dance
   E) Track

QUESTIONS: Disorders of Cognition, Language & Learning

330) Which of the following is true regarding hearing impairment in children?

   A) All newborns should be screened for hearing loss at 9 months of age
   B) Infants who exhibit language related milestones including cooing, pointing and social smiling are unlikely to have a hearing deficit
   C) Early intervention services should be implemented at two years of age
   D) Newborns who fail their hearing screen should have a comprehensive audiological evaluation by 3 months of age.
   E) Auditory communication is favorable to sign language for language development

331) You are evaluating a child during a well exam and can understand around half of what she is trying to communicate. This would be considered average language development for which aged child?

   A) 12 months
   B) 24 months
   C) 36 months
   D) 48 months
   E) 60 months

332) You are evaluating a 4 year old boy whose family immigrated from Nicaragua one year ago. Spanish is the primary language spoken at home but he has been attending daycare where English is spoken and he speaks and understands both languages. However, he does seem to have difficulty hearing and saying words in Spanish, and English words that begin contain the letter S or F, and English words that have a th sound. The most likely explanation for this would be?

   A) Bilingual language delay
   B) Social anxiety
   C) Hearing deficit
   D) Autism spectrum disorder
   E) Normal language development

Behavior and Mental Health

333) Each of the following would be appropriate management of a teenager who is otherwise healthy but has been showing signs of moderate fatigue and expressing dark thoughts. Her physical exam is unremarkable and she denies any suicidal thoughts or intentions. There is a family history of depression. Which of the following would be an appropriate initial step:

   A) Review of nutrition and exercise
   B) Complete blood count
   C) Thyroid studies
   D) Psychiatric consultation
   E) Start fluoxetine

334) Which of the following is true regarding he association of tics and stimulant medication?

   A) Stimulant medications lower the threshold for developing tics
   B) Stimulant medications must be discontinued until the tics resolve
   C) Nonstimulant medications such as atomoxetine are indicated when tics continue after a 2nd trial of stimulants
   D) Stimulant medications are a common cause of tics
   E) Tics are not associated with stimulant medication use

335) Regarding stimulant medication for attention deficit hyperactivity disorder (ADHD) which of the following is true?

   A) Dosing is weight dependent
   B) Patients should always start with short-acting rather than long-acting medications
   C) Baseline labs and EKG should be done routinely
   D) If normative functioning is obtained, behavioral-modification therapy may not be indicated
   E) If one stimulant fails to work, it is unlikely that another one will work

QUESTIONS: Psychosocial

336) Which of the following methods of psychotherapy is considered to be the most effective in treating mild forms of depression in teenagers?

   A) Long term Freudian psychoanalysis
   B) Individual psychodynamic therapy
   C) Cognitive behavioral therapy
   D) School based intervention
   E) Peer to Peer file sharing therapy

337) Which of the following medications is approved for treating depression in children 8 years and older?

   A) Fluoxetine
   B) Fluvoxamine
   C) Citalopram
   D) Escitalopram
   E) Sertraline

Psychosocial

338) His mother, a VP for a venture capital group, brings Johnny Edhopperman to your ER. You are in the middle of your 89-hour shift in central Connecticut. Mom is exasperated because her child has been vomiting for 6 months and none of the doctors who work in "the City" have done anything.

   The mother calmly tells you to "look at my son; he is clearly hypovolemic, dry and his cap refill is 3 seconds or more. Please help him." After obtaining electrolytes and giving him several normal saline boluses, which additional studies should you order to clinch the diagnosis for this mother?

   A) Maternal porcelain levels
   B) Serum emetine levels
   C) No labs. Ask the mother to prepare a press release since the workup was all wrong and the public needs to know
   D) CBC, Diff, Blood Culture and ESR
   E) Abdominal and head MRIs

339) In the following set of questions, decide if each numbered choice applies to (A) only, (B) only, both (C), or neither (D):

1) First third of the night
2) Enuresis
3) Mobile during episode
4) Recall of episode
5) Positive family history

(A) Night terrors
(B) Nightmares
(C) Both
(D) Neither

340) An 8-year-old boy with ADHD is brought in for routine evaluation. His parents want to know about appropriate dietary therapy. Which of the following is the BEST advice based upon the latest research?

A) Restrict all foods that contain sugar
B) Eliminate all foods that contain artificial coloring and artificial preservatives
C) Eliminate all processed foods
D) Start a guten-free diet
E) Eat a well balanced diet; ADHD has no relation to diet

341) A 2-1/2-year-old boy is brought to your office for a routine visit. The parents notice that he will often repeat the first word in a sentence, especially when he is rushed or tired. Although it doesn't occur all the time, it does occur when the child is asked a question. You should:

A) Order a neurological workup
B) Obtain a formal hearing evaluation
C) Refer the child for speech therapy
D) Rule out ankyloglossia
E) Reassure the mother

QUESTIONS: Psychosocial

342) Which of the following would be reasonable expectations of a child with an IQ of 70?

A) Achieve academic skill at the high school level
B) Some vocational skills while living at a supervised group home
C) Marry and become a successful parent
D) Need assistance with self-help skills
E) Become a political pundit on their own show Sunday mornings on major network

343) The most common presentation of intellectual disability is:

A) Delayed motor development
B) Poor social skills
C) Reading disability
D) Language delay
E) Seizures

344) Each one of the following is a true statement regarding primitive reflexes EXCEPT:

A) They are normal in infants but abnormal in others
B) They are brainstem-mediated
C) They disappear during the first year as voluntary motor activity emerges
D) Corneal reflex is an example
E) They are never normal in adult males

345) An 18-month-old former 24-week premie is being seen for a routine well-baby visit. The child was ventilator-dependent for one month, with head ultrasounds, hearing screens, and eye exams all normal. The mother is concerned because of the lack of speech development. You note that the baby seems to respond to a one-step verbal command and can wave goodbye. She uses one-syllable words to express herself in addition to *dada* and *mama*. You should:

A) Reassure the mother
B) Head CT to rule out any head bleed that was missed initially
C) Repeat the hearing test
D) Refer to a speech pathologist
E) She is past the time when prematurity would account for the delay

346) You need to evaluate an 18 month old boy because his parents are concerned about his tendency to bang his head and suck his thumb especially before going to bed. His growth and development are otherwise normal.

The most likely diagnosis is

A) Tourette Syndrome
B) Rett syndrome
C) Pervasive developmental disorder
D) Autism
E) Normal developmental variant

347) The parents of a 9-year-old boy report being awakened by a panicky scream coming from their child's room roughly 2 hours after he fell asleep. They were unable to console him or wake him up. When they arrived in his room he was tachycardic and tachypneic and he eventually calmed down. He was unable to recall the event in the morning. You should advise them that this is MOST likely due to:

A) Watching American idol earlier
B) Nightmare
C) Night terror
D) Rolandic epilepsy
E) Anxiety disorder

QUESTIONS: Psychosocial

348) An 8-year-old child is brought to your practice because of his inability to "stay on task" at school and his banter with the kids in the back of the room where he sits. When asked what the problem is, he tells you *"I'm sorry I wasn't listening".* The parents state there is nothing wrong and all he needs is a tutor.

They note that his dad, a trader on the NY stock exchange making millions had the same difficulty when he was a child. Your BEST approach to the problem is:

A) Ask dad if he would be willing to train you to work on the floor of the exchange as his protégé.
B) Explain that the beneficial effects of stimulant meds are almost immediate, and write a script for 5 mg methylphenidate q AM with followup in one week.
C) Explain that the beneficial effects of stimulant meds are evident, and write a script for 5 mg methylphenidate q AM for 3 days followed by 10 mg dexmethylphenidate XR q day if it is working, with followup in a week.
D) Explain the possibility of a diagnosis of ADD and that the diagnosis does not carry a poor prognosis. Offer literature on the subject and suggest a followup visit in a week.
E) Write a script for methylphenidate 5 mg, schedule an appointment for psychological testing to rule out a learning disorder, and suggest that he be seated in the front of the room where there is less distraction.

349) A 7-year-old boy is evaluated because of a recent deterioration in school performance. Medical history is unremarkable except for hydronephrosis with associated infection for which he received a 1-month course of aminoglycoside therapy 6 months ago. Which of the following is the most likely cause of this boy's academic problems?

A) Focal brain abscess
B) Progressive uremia
C) ADHD
D) Temporal lobe seizures
E) Hearing loss

350) An infant sits comfortably on your examining table. He takes a stick from your hand, and transfers it to his other hand. His mother reports that he crawls. He does not pull himself to a standing position, but he supports his weight and takes tentative and clumsy steps with both hands held. The developmental age of this infant is closest to:

A) 6 months
B) 9 months
C) 12 months
D) 15 months
E) 18 months

351) An 11-year-old boy is being evaluated because his teachers do not think that his school performance matches his ability. His birth history is normal.

His teachers report that he leaves his seat at inappropriate times and talks excessively during class. The parents assume that their son will eventually outgrow this "adjustment period".

His school performance has declined steadily for the past 2 years, which his teachers attribute to difficulty completing assignments and homework. General physical findings are normal. The boy is well behaved but fidgety. Neurologic evaluation is normal. He has well-coordinated gross and fine motor movements.

When you evaluate him he focuses well and pays attention. Which of the following is the most likely diagnosis?

A) Oppositional defiant disorder
B) Mental retardation
C) Gilles de la Tourette syndrome
D) Normal developmental period
E) Attention deficit hyperactivity disorder

QUESTIONS: Psychosocial

352) You are evaluating a 2 year old for a well visit. The mother is a single mother, there during her lunch hour and is breast feeding her 6 month old. Her 4 year old other child is in the waiting room playing. The mother had to go out several times to attend to the 4 year old who was fighting with another child in the waiting room play area.

She is awaiting the arrival of their part time nanny who takes over at lunch. The mother works out of their home office and watches the patient and their other two children while working out of her home office as a paralegal.

What would you suggest for this mother?

A) Offer her additional work as a paralegal
B) Refer her for social work consultation
C) Suggest that she work at night
D) Suggest that she incorporate the 4 year old into her work routine
E) That she is doing a fine job juggling her responsibilities.

353) Each of the following is true regarding families with a child with a chronic illness *except:*

A) Children with special needs are at increased risk for physical abuse and neglect at home
B) Children with special needs are at increased risk for physical abuse and neglect in educational and child care settings
C) The divorce rate is the same as in families without a child with a special need
D) Family members are at increased risk for depression
E) Parents who are health professionals do not necessarily cope better than do parents who are not health professionals.

354) Which of the following is the most likely explanation for a 6 week old infant who cries 3 hours a day most days every week? The crying occurs suddenly, is persistent, does not respond to feeding or changing, and has been going on since the infant was 2 weeks of age. Her growth and development are normal.

A) The need to change formula
B) The need for the breastfeeding mother to monitor her diet closely
C) Infantile colic
D) Intussusception
E) Reflux esophagitis

355) Which of the following is true regarding TV watching in children?

   A) More than 50% of parents enforce TV viewing limits
   B) Less than 50% of homes of children 8 years and older have the TV on during meals
   C) Only 25% of children 8 years and older have video game systems in their room
   D) Only 25% of children 8 years and older have TVs in their rooms
   E) The AAP recommends that children younger than 2 years of age should watch no TV

356) Which of the following is most effective in pediatric patients requiring pharmacological treatment of separation anxiety disorder?

   A) Desipramine
   B) Atomoxetine
   C) Fluoxetine
   D) Clonazepam
   E) Risperidone

Critical Care

357) All of the following interfere with the accuracy of pulse oximetry EXCEPT:

   A) Methemoglobinemia
   B) Elevated carboxyhemoglobin
   C) Impaired perfusion
   D) Hypoglycemia
   E) Hypothermia

QUESTIONS: Critical Care

358) Match the diagnoses on the left with the arterial blood gas results on the right:

			pH	PCO$_2$	Bicarb
1)	Respiratory acidosis	(A)	7.25	24	10
2)	Respiratory alkalosis	(B)	7.62	22	37
3)	Metabolic alkalosis	(C)	7.25	60	38
4)	Metabolic acidosis	(D)	7.01	62	12
5)	Respiratory acidosis (compensated)	(E)	7.52	18	10
6)	Respiratory alkalosis (compensated)	(F)	7.36	20	10
7)	Combined acidosis (metabolic – respiratory)	(G)	7.52	34	37
8)	Combined alkalosis (metabolic – respiratory)	(H)	7.36	65	40

359) Which of the children below could be safely discharged from the ER and observed at home after a near-drowning episode?

A) A child with a brief generalized seizure
B) Child who required CPR in the field who is now stable with a GCS of 15
C) Child submerged less than one minute who received no CPR in the field
D) Child who was stable but is now tachypneic
E) Child who initially aspirated water but is now stable

360) Which of following statements regarding *hyperventilation syndrome* is true?

A) It is always caused by a *panic attack*
B) It is breathing in excess of metabolic requirements resulting in hypercapnia
C) The safest treatment in the acute setting is breathing into a paper bag
D) When anxiety is the cause, reassurance will often resolve the problem
E) The absence of chest pain or fever rules out congestive heart failure and pneumonia

361) You are treating a 12 month old child who is febrile, tachypneic, and moderately hypotensive with scattered petechiae on the trunk and purpuric lesions on the ankles. Until a definitive diagnosis is established which of the following would be the most appropriate treatment?

A) Referral to child protective services for child abuse and neglect
B) Assume a diagnosis of Henoch Schönlein purpura and observe overnight
C) IV Ceftriaxone
D) IV Vancomycin
E) IV Vancomycin and Ceftriaxone

Emergency Medicine

362) With regards to sexual abuse, which of the following is true?

A) A normal genito-anal exam all but rules out sexual abuse
B) A crescentic hymen on physical exam is pathognomonic for sexual assault
C) Labial adhesions are most commonly caused by repeated sexual abuse
D) Posterior hymenal tears on vaginal exam are more consistent with sexual abuse
E) Physical exam should focus on the labia majora for signs of abuse

363) Which of the following is the most appropriate location for insertion of an intraosseous needle?

A) Midpoint of the tibial shaft
B) Midpoint of the femoral shaft, in the midline
C) 1 cm proximal to the tibial tuberosity
D) Anteromedial tibia, 2 cm distal to the tuberosity
E) Mid sternum

QUESTIONS: Emergency Medicine

364) Match the cause of abdominal pain on the left with the clinical descriptions on the right.

1) Ureteropelvic junction obstructions
2) Dysmenorrhea
3) Acute intermittent porphyria
4) Psychogenic abdominal pain (conversion disorder)

(A) Labile 13 year old with a depressed parent
(B) Paroxysmal abdominal pain along with headaches, dizziness and syncope
(C) Painless bloody diarrhea
(D) Cramping, dull, midline pain
(E) Recurrent episodes of periumbilical and midepigastric cramps with episodic vomiting

365) Which of the following is the MOST appropriate initial treatment of severe hypertension in a known asthmatic?

A) Benzodiazepines
B) Morphine
C) epinephrine
D) Vasodilators
E) Beta-blockers

366) An 18 year-old comatose boy is brought to the ER. The friend who accompanied him to the ER states he noticed that the patient took a small fistful of some pills earlier, but knows of no other history. Temperature is 37.2 C, heart rate is 45/min, RR is 6/min, and BP is 75/45 mm Hg. Pupils are 1.0 mm in diameter. There is no nystagmus or spontaneous lacrimation. The patient is responsive only to deep painful stimuli and is hyporeflexic. Ingestion of which of the following substances is MOST likely?

A) Diphenhydramine
B) Tricyclic antidepressants
C) Organophosphates
D) Methylphenidate
E) Opiates

367) You are evaluating an *afebrile* 3-year-old boy who will not bear weight. You order x-ray studies of the lower extremities,[11] which show no evidence of any fractures. The MOST appropriate next step to look for occult fractures would be:

A) A conventional CT scan
B) Technetium bone scan
C) A skeletal survey
D) MRI
E) PET scan

368) The reduction of intracranial pressure following the IV administration of mannitol to patients with cerebral edema is caused by decrease in:

A) Cerebral volume
B) Brain water volume
C) CSF volume
D) Cardiac output
E) Respiratory rate

369) A 5-year-old boy was found in the family swimming pool and was resuscitated on-site by EMS. He arrives at the ER in minimal respiratory distress with vital signs stable. He is hospitalized and becomes tachypneic over the next 18 hours.

The initial chest x-ray demonstrated a fine reticular infiltrate. A second x-ray taken later shows evidence of pulmonary edema. Clinically, the oxygen saturations decrease and he requires oxygen, and you note audible crackles. The respiratory distress increases and you intubate and start the child on mechanical ventilation. Which of the following would BEST explain the deteriorating status?

A) Poor initial resuscitation
B) Tension pneumothorax
C) Pulmonary embolism
D) Acute respiratory distress syndrome
E) Aspiration pneumonia

---

[11] Known as "legs" to the rest of the world.

370) A 3-year-old with a history of bloody diarrhea and a high fever is in your waiting room. A frantic pharmaceutical rep (who dropped his box of donuts covered with promotional stickers because the child is having a generalized seizure) calls you out. You step over and onto some of the donuts and realize you must:

A) Ask for new donuts
B) Administer 3% Normal Saline
C) Start antibiotics for *E. coli* O157:H7
D) Treat for *Salmonella* once the seizure is brought under control
E) Treat for *Shigella* once the seizure is brought under control

371) You would be correct in making a presumptive diagnosis of child abuse in each of the following situations EXCEPT:

A) A 4-year-old with evenly distributed purpuric lesions on the lower extremities
B) Fracture of the posterior ribs following a fall from a chair
C) A 6-year-old with several fractures in different stages who has otherwise been doing well
D) A 2-year-old hyperactive child with a fracture noted on the sternum of the chest
E) A 6-year-old with a spiral fracture on the mid shaft of the humerus

372) A 6-year-old is brought to the emergency department after being struck by a car driven by a driver talking on a cell phone.[12] He presents with abdominal tenderness, decreased bowel sounds, and some guarding, but no rebound tenderness. Your INITIAL step should be:

A) Abdominal plain film
B) Abdominal ultrasound
C) Airway assessment
D) Evaluate cap refill while preparing for IV placement and intraosseous line if necessary
E) Computed tomography

---

[12] The driver is brought in moments later with "cell phone impaled tympanic membrane syndrome."

373) Regarding the physical abuse of children which of the following is true?

   A) Minor injuries do not represent a pattern of abuse
   B) The age of a bruise can always be determined by the color
   C) Bruises from accidental injury can be identified by location.
   D) Cultural healing practices that leave skin marks have not been well described
   E) Burn marks in a splash pattern are typically a result of deliberate abuse

374) A 20-year-old student has an injured arm. X-ray study of the distal humerus reveals a fracture in the supracondylar region. Which of the following is the most concerning complication of such an injury?

   A) Neurovascular compromise
   B) Growth plate injury
   C) Fat embolism
   D) Pulmonary embolism
   E) Hypercalcemia secondary to immobilization

375) One hour ago a 10-year-old boy was a passenger in an automobile that was involved in a collision. The child was wearing a lap belt and did not lose consciousness. He now has abdominal pain but no headache.

   The patient is well oriented and alert. Physical exam reveals no evidence of bone fractures. There is mild bruising where the lap belt crossed the abdomen, and the abdomen is tender throughout. Lab studies reveal a HGB of 9.0 g/dL and a HCT of 27%. You suspect that the patient has a ruptured spleen.

   Which of the following would be the *most appropriate* next step in confirming the diagnosis?

   A) CT of the abdomen with IV contrast
   B) US of the abdomen
   C) CT of the abdomen without contrast
   D) Paracentesis
   E) Serial HCT determinations

QUESTIONS: Emergency Medicine

376) Which of the following would be the most important initial step when assessing a fallen football player with a potential cervical spine injury?

   A) Remove the helmet
   B) Remove the facemask
   C) Palpate the cervical spine for tenderness
   D) Assess the airway
   E) Assess the mechanism of injury

377) Which of the following is true regarding ankle injuries?

   A) Improper shoes and poor training are the most common causes of ankle injury
   B) Fracture the 1st metatarsal is commonly seen with inversion injuries
   C) With a minor injury with no point tenderness or limping , ankle mobilization can proceed within 18 hours
   D) Rest, ice, compression and elevation is most helpful for 48 hours after the ankle injury
   E) Heat should be applied to the injury initially along with elevation

378) Which of the following is true regarding fentanyl in conscious sedation ?

   A) Fentanyl has a longer half-life than morphine
   B) Provides sufficient anxiolysis to be used without other agents
   C) If titrated too rapidly can result in chest wall stiffness
   D) It is indicated for non-painful prolonged distressing procedures
   E) Has no role in conscious sedation in children

379) Each of the following would be helpful nonpharmacological methods to reduce anxiety during painful procedures performed in children *except*:

   A) Cartoons
   B) Breathing exercises
   C) Video games
   D) Reassuring comments such as "I'm sorry we have to do this"
   E) Music

380) 90 % of allergic reactions to food are due to the following *except*:

A) Strawberries
B) Milk
C) Eggs
D) Soy
E) Fish

381) You are evaluating a previously healthy 4 year old who presents to the emergency department with a 1 day history of paroxysmal coughing and posttussive forceful emesis. He was brought to the ER because of 2 episodes of emesis that were blood streaked. The physical exam is unremarkable including the absence of any significant abdominal pain or wheeze , rales or rhonchi.

The most likely explanation for the clinical presentation would be:

A) Inexplicable
B) Acute alcohol intoxication
C) Mallory Weiss Tear
D) Peptic Ulcer disease
E) Gastritis

382) Each of the following is true regarding cyclic vomiting syndrome *except:*

A) Amitriptyline and propranolol are effective during acute episodes
B) Intervals of normal health is typical between episodes
C) 3 or more episodes of recurrent vomiting is part of the diagnosis
D) No lab results to support an alternative diagnosis
E) No radiographic evidence to support an alternative diagnosis

Pharmacology and Pain Management

383) In the following set of questions, for each numbered word or phrase, choose the lettered heading that is MOST CLOSELY ASSOCIATED with it. Lettered headings may be selected once, more than once, or not at all.

1) Metabolic acidosis
2) Hypokalemic alkalosis
3) Contraction alkalosis
4) Potassium sparing

(A) Furosemide
(B) Acetazolamide
(C) Spironolactone
(D) Hydrochlorothiazide

384) Trimethoprim/ Sulfamethoxazole would be the first line treatment for each of the following EXCEPT :

A) Pneumocystis carinii pneumonia prophylaxis
B) Urinary tract infection prophylaxis
C) Urinary tract infection due to enterococcus
D) Listeria monocytogenes in penicillin allergic patients
E) Exacerbation of chronic bronchitis

385) Which of the following supplements should be used with caution when taking sedatives?

A) Echinacea
B) Ginseng
C) Valerian Root
D) St. John's Wort
E) Peppermint Patty

386) Which of the following medications is postulated to act by inhibiting serotonin reuptake?

   A) Echinacea
   B) Ginseng
   C) St. Johns' Wort
   D) Valerian Root
   E) St. John's Band

387) Match each chemotherapeutic agent on the left to its associated *toxicity* on the right.

   1) Cyclophosphamide   (A) Cardiac toxicity
   2) Bleomycin   (B) CNS problems
   3) Doxorubicin   (C) Hemorrhagic cystitis
   4) Anthracycline   (D) Neurotoxicity
   5) Vincristine   (E) Oral ulcerations
   6) Asparaginase   (F) Pancreatitis
   7) Methotrexate   (G) Pulmonary fibrosis

Research and Statistics

388) Each of the following is true regarding *descriptive epidemiological studies* except:

   A) They use surveys, surveillance reports, and cross sectional analysis
   B) They describe patterns of disease
   C) They followup on case reports
   D) They test predefined hypotheses
   E) They help define a hypothesis for further study

QUESTIONS: Research and Statistics

389) Which of the following formulas reflects the sensitivity of a lab test?

TP = True Positive
FN = False negatives
TN = True negatives

A) $\dfrac{TP}{TP + FN}$

B) $\dfrac{FN}{TP + FN}$

C) $\dfrac{TN}{TN + FP}$

D) $\dfrac{FP}{TN + FP}$

E) $\dfrac{TP}{TP + FP}$

390) Which of the following formula reflects the specificity of a lab test?

TP = True Positive
FN = False negatives
TN = True negatives

A) $\dfrac{TP}{TP + FN}$

B) $\dfrac{FN}{TP + FN}$

C) $\dfrac{TN}{TN + FP}$

D) $\dfrac{FP}{TN + FP}$

E) $\dfrac{TP}{TP + FP}$

391) Case reports play an important role in medical research and the advancement of knowledge in each of the following ways *except*:

A) They help identify correlations between two events
B) They help identify rare adverse events
C) They establish causation of rare adverse events
D) They can help identify emerging health situations that require investigation
E) They can provide clues regarding events causing disease

392) Each of the following is true regarding prospective cohort studies *except*:

A) It is not good for studying diseases with long latency periods
B) It is an excellent method to study risk factors for rare diseases
C) It can be expensive and time consuming
D) Differential loss to followup can introduce a bias
E) It requires a large number of subjects studied over a long period of time

393) An investigator compares the results of laboratory tests with the presence of a disease and tabulates the results as follows:

Test Results	With Disease	Without Disease
Positive	81	5
Negative	37	48

The investigator reports that 0.68 is the:

A) Sensitivity of the test
B) Specificity of the test
C) Prevalence of the disease
D) Accuracy of the test
E) Positive predictive value for the test

QUESTIONS: Research and Statistics

394) An investigator compares the results of laboratory testing with the presence of a disease and tabulates the results as follows:

Test Results	With Disease	Without Disease
Positive	81	5
Negative	37	48

The investigator reports that 0.90 is the:

A) Sensitivity of the test
B) Specificity of the test
C) Prevalence of the disease
D) Accuracy of the test
E) Positive predictive value for the test

395) An investigator compares the results of laboratory testing with the presence of a disease and tabulates the results as follows:

Test Results	With Disease	Without Disease
Positive	81	5
Negative	37	48

The investigator reports that 0.94 is the:

A) Sensitivity of the test
B) Specificity of the test
C) Prevalence of the disease
D) Accuracy of the test
E) Positive predictive value for the test

Copyright 2018 Medhumor Medical Publications, LLC

Ethics for Primary Care Physicians

396) You are working with the family of a child with end stage liver disease. They read on Reddit® about lime in the coconut therapy that is available south of the border, way south of the border. What is the proper response to their query?

   A) If it is not supported by research, you don't want to know about it
   B) You support what the family feels is in their best interests
   C) You will explore and discuss what you discover with the family
   D) By definition, such treatment constitutes nonmaleficence
   E) By definition, such treatment is inconsistent with the duty for beneficence

397) Which of the following is true regarding palliative care in children?

   A) Palliative care is beneficial exclusively to cancer patients
   B) Palliative care is beneficial to those children at or near the end of their lives
   C) Palliative care is primarily focused on helping families cope with life threatening conditions
   D) Families must make a choice between palliative and cure-directed treatment
   E) Palliative treatment often means forgoing life extending treatments

398) The father of one of your patients bursts into the waiting area. You overhear him complaining about the fact that he received a bill from the previous visit last week due to his having a high in-network deductible. The staff quietly settles the matter. A few minutes later, in front of his 16 year old son, your patient, he insists that you "drug test" his son who he is sure is using drugs and "other stuff". The most appropriate next step would be to:

   A) Go into a tirade about your opinion on the Affordable Care Act
   B) Drug test the father
   C) Drug test the patient but only if he agrees
   D) Drug test the patient with or without his consent since he is under 18
   E) Speak with the boy confidentially to review the situation

QUESTIONS: Ethics for Primary Care Physicians

399) Which of the following is consistent with American Academy of Pediatric guidelines regarding expert testimony in court for medical malpractice cases?

   A) Testifying outside ones area of expertise can result in suspension of your license to practice medicine
   B) Testimony should be based on one's experience in similar situations
   C) Compensation based on a sliding scale based on the amount of awarded judgement is now considered the fairest method to gauge appropriate compensation
   D) It is never appropriate to spend the majority of time solely as an expert witness
   E) Pediatricians have an ethical and professional duty to assist in the administration of justice in civil and court proceedings

400) You correctly diagnosed a teenager in the early stages of meningococcemia. He was in the Bender-Duster Left Wing pavilion ICU for 4 days and has recovered completely. The parents tell you that they didn't realize at the time the morbidity and mortality rate is well over 60% and they cannot thank you enough. They offer you season tickets for the local NHL game, are worth $10,000, since they know you are an avid hockey fan. You refuse, but they insist that you at least let them know which games you wish to attend. Which of the following would be the most appropriate way to handle this situation?

   A) Let them know that you will be glad to take them up on the offer as long as the patient attends the games with you
   B) Ask them for 20 separate gift cards worth $500 so you are not over the $500 maximal ethical limit for patient gifts
   C) Have them make a donation to the Bender Duster Pavilion as a token of their gratitude to you and your staff
   D) Have them give the tickets to your friend Joey since you cannot accept a direct gift
   E) Let them know that you cannot accept any gifts or donations

Patient Safety and Quality Improvement

401) Each of the following is true regarding *near miss events* <u>except</u> :

A) A near miss event can be intercepted
B) A near miss event can be non-intercepted
C) A non-intercepted near miss event always results in harm to the patient
D) A near miss event can be a result of incorrect keyboard entry into an EMR
E) A near miss event is a potential adverse event which placed patient at significant risk of injury

402) Each of the following is true regarding patient safety in the pediatric setting except:

A) Adverse events occur in 1% of pediatric hospitalizations
B) 60% of pediatric adverse events are preventable
C) The rising rate of adverse drug events may be due to the increased ability to detect them rather than increased actual incidence
D) The risk for adverse drug events is 3 times higher in adult hospitalized patients than in children
E) Traditional or folk remedies can have harmful interactions with standard medications

403) Which of the following is a true statement regarding medical errors in the outpatient pediatric setting?

A) Template based e-prescribing increases the risk for medication error
B) The level of parental education does not affect the frequency of dosing errors in the home
C) Readily available household measuring spoons are adequate for medication administration
D) Over immunization is a common error when multiple clinicians are involved in the immunization of a child
E) Medical errors in the ambulatory setting is limited to medication and immunization errors

QUESTIONS: Patient Safety and Quality Improvement

404) Which of the following is true regarding patient safety during transition of care from one team to another?

A) Performing sign out at the bedside with patient and parental involvement increases risk for error
B) Limitation on resident physician work hours has resulted in reduced fatigue and less patient continuity
C) Standardization of transition communication can result in increased miscommunication
D) Communication errors are the root cause of less than 10 % of sentinel events
E) Limitations on resident physician work hours has reduced fatigue and better patient continuity

405) It's Friday afternoon at 5:15 PM and you just went back to your office to make sure you locked your door and the phone rings. You are looking forward to a weekend of hiking and golf with Phil a visiting medical school classmate. It is CB-Ess pharmacy on the line. Your patient, Charlie B is here for his methadone prescription. The pharmacist wants to verify the prescription before dispensing it. You recall sending in a prescription for Ritalin®, since Charlie is being treated for ADHD. This is most likely due to or could be described as a:

A) Prank phone call from Phil trying to pry you out of the office
B) Near miss intercepted event
C) Drug seeker who hacked into your system
D) Near miss non intercepted event
E) Adverse drug event

Answers

ANSWERS: Growth and Development

Growth and Development

1) **A)** In the not so distant past, the appropriate management for failure to thrive was hospital admission and observation of feeding and growing. . If the child gained weight in such an environment, feeding and other maternal-child issues would be identified. Routine labs were also considered to be an appropriate first step. This is no longer the case. Therefore for the patient in the vignette, Choice A, which indicates inpatient evaluation, would not be considered to be an appropriate initial intervention.

   Occupational therapy would be considered appropriate in evaluating feeding practices. Social services and behavioral therapy would be appropriate in evaluating psychosocial issues. Clearly evaluating nutritional causes of failure to thrive on an outpatient basis would be very appropriate.

2) **C)** The World Health Organization (WHO) growth charts are based on infants who were exclusively breast-fed until 4 months of age and continued to be breast fed until 1 year of age. Therefore, the WHO growth charts reflect "ideal growth" and should be used to assess growth of children younger than 2 years of age. The US Center for Disease Control (CDC) growth charts correlate with optimal growth in *formula* fed infants. Height at 2 **years** of age correlates well with mean parental height.

3) **E** Both renal dialysis and renal transplantation improve growth but do **not** allow for catchup growth. Improved nutrition and supplementation do result in improved linear growth rates.

   On the other hand metabolic bone disease can occur with chronic kidney disease resulting in impaired linear growth. Prolonged steroid use decreases growth hormone secretion and liver production of IGF-1 both decreasing growth.

   Questions on growth hormone and insulin growth factor-1 (IGF-1) can be tricky depending on what is asked. While it is true that chronic steroid use can decrease the secretion of both of these crucial hormones, in general decreased levels are not the explanation of decreased growth with chronic renal disease.

It is true that "abnormalities" of GH and IGF-1 result in gross failure. However GH levels sometimes are actually elevated. It is the **resistance or insensitivity** that is the cause of decreased growth. Regarding IGF-1 it is the decreased **bioactivity, due to increased IGF binding proteins** that cause the growth failure.

Be careful how such questions might be phrased!

An additional contributor to the growth failure is anemia due to decreased erythropoietin. Erythropoietin supplementation can help improve linear growth rates.

4) E) The Pediatric Symptom Checklist (PSC) is a general mental health disorder screening tool, valid for patients between the ages of 6 – 16 years of age.

The Patient Health Questionnaire (PHQ-9) is a depression rating scale for adults and adolescents. It is not a general mental health condition screening tool.

The Child Behavior Checklist is a mental health screening tool that is used by mental health clinics and is too complicated and convoluted to be used as a screen in the general pediatric office setting.

The Ages and Stages Questionnaire® (ASQ) is a general developmental screen with several age appropriate versions. It is valid through age 3.

The LMAO Scale (Lexington Mental Agility Online) is there for comic effect we just made it up to be consistent with our "Laughing Your Way To Passing the Pediatric Boards"® theme.

5) C) Weight or height greater than 85th or 90th percentiles (answers A and D) in and of themselves would not be considered sufficient in determining a 2 year old is at high risk for obesity since they may be appropriate for his height.

However a BMI of greater than 85th percentile is by definition overweight and would be considered to be a significant risk factor to warrant monitoring the child and try to prevent obesity from occurring. Therefore choice C is correct.

Large for gestational age (LGA) infants may be due to large parents genetically or to large mothers due to diabetes. They certainly warrant close observation, but are not necessarily at high risk for obesity based solely on their LGA status.

Nutrition

6) **E)** Breast-feeding should continue through 12 months of age if possible. This is a trick choice because the AAP suggests *exclusive* breast-feeding throughout the first 6 months. Therefore "breast-feeding through the first 6 months is adequate" is not really a true statement since additional breast feeding through the first year would be more appropriate.

The components of breast milk are **not** constant at all during the first year. The components change to coincide with the nutritional needs during the first year. Breast milk contains **IgA** not IgG. This is another instance where reading the question carefully is crucial. At casual glance it is very easy to confuse IgA with IgG.

Human milk does **not** contain T cells and alpha interferon; however, there is strong evidence that breast milk complements the infant's own immune system via immunomodulation.

7) **D)** Phylloquinone, fluoride, vitamin D, and vitamin B12 can be found in breast milk under *most* conditions. However, of the choices listed, only ascorbic acid (vitamin C) can be found in adequate amounts under *all* conditions.

Phylloquinone is also known as **vitamin K**.[1] Initially infants, even exclusively breast-fed babies, are at risk for vitamin K deficiency. These infants are therefore not good at producing vitamin K dependent factors (remember 2, 7, 9, and 10).

Exclusively breast-fed infants are also at risk for being vitamin D deficient if the mother is not getting adequate vitamin D in her diet and/or the infant is not getting adequate sun exposure.

As for fluoride, **it IS found in breast milk**, *if there are adequate amounts in the water supply*.

Therefore this would not be the case if the mother is drinking well water or other sources that do not contain flouride.

However, it is important to note that the AAP recommends fluoride supplementation for infants over 6 months who are exclusively breast fed and are not getting fluoridated water.

For all you strict vegetarians out there, remember to take B12 supplements. Vegetarians are at risk for being **B12 deficient** and therefore will not be providing enough in their breast milk if they are not taking B12 supplements.

---

[1] Remember to commit these fancier names to memory; they will employ anything to get you into the wrong side of passing.

8) 1) (C)
    2) (D)
    3) (B)
    4) (A)
    5) (A)

If freedom's just another word for "nothing left to lose" then ergocalciferol is just another name for Vitamin D_2 (it has TWO Cs) and cholecalciferol is just another name for Vitamin D_3 (it has THREE Cs).

25, hydroxy vitamin D is hydroxylated in the liver. The first group (-25) is added in the liver because there is only one liver.

1, 25 hydroxy vitamin D is activated calcitriol and hydroxylated in the kidney.

The active final product has two added groups (-25 and then -1) and is finalized in the kidneys because there are two kidneys.

9) 1) (C)
    2) (A)
    3) (B)

Essential fatty acid deficiency can result in → scaly dermatitis, alopecia, thrombocytopenia

Zinc deficiency can result in → dry skin, poor wound healing, perioral rash

Vitamin E deficiency can result in → hemolytic anemia, peripheral edema, thrombocytopenia

Ascorbic acid deficiency (scurvy) presents with bleeding gums, leg tenderness and poor wound healing.

10) B) In "developed" countries such as the United States where the endemic rate of HIV infection is low and commercially available formula is a safer alternative, breast-feeding would be contraindicated, as would the use of pooled breast milk.

However, in "developing countries" outside the US where HIV is more endemic, severe poverty more common, and commercially available formula not as readily available, the risks of "not breast-feeding" and the subsequent risks of inadequate malnutrition may outweigh the risks against contracting the HIV virus from breast milk. That would be a more complicated question.

However this question is specific regarding protocol in the United States where safe alternatives to breast-feeding are available.

ANSWERS: Nutrition

11) B) Medium chain triglycerides (MCT) *are* present in human milk and *some* infant formula.

However medium chain triglycerides are <u>not present in cow's milk</u>. They do <u>not</u> require micelle formation with bile salts for adequate absorption; this makes MCTs a good source of rapidly available metabolic fuel.

12) A) Biotin deficiency results primarily in dermatitis, and more specifically seborrhea. You can picture a "rusty **tin**" to remember that **biotin** causes skin problems to lock this into memory.

13) B) Oxaluria, the excretion of excessive amounts of calcium oxalate, can result from excessive intake of ascorbic acid or vitamin C.

Ascorbic acid taken in excessive dosages can also lead to nephrocalcinosis.

The water soluble vitamins are all the Bs (including Biotin) and Vitamin C.

14) D) The water soluble vitamins are all the Bs (including Biotin) and Vitamin C. You would need to know that ***cobalamin*** is the formal name for ***vitamin B12***, which is commonly deficient in a vegetarian diet. This concept is frequently tested on the exam.

It can also be an issue with a **breast-feeding mother** who is on a vegetarian diet. Vitamin B12 deficiency often results in megaloblastic anemia.

15) C) The clinical description is of a child suffering from retinol or vitamin A deficiency. Bumping into objects at night would be consistent with night blindness (nyctalopia). The silvery patches on the eye are known as bitot spots which is also consistent with Vitamin A deficiency.

To avoid permanent blindness retinol supplementation is crucial.

16) E) The best explanation for *all* of the clinical findings in this patient would be Cystic fibrosis.

Cystic fibrosis would explain repeated bouts of bronchiolitis as well as the foul smelling diarrhea which would be due to malabsorption.

Malabsorption would lead absorption of fat soluble vitamins. These would include Vitamin D deficiency which would explain the low serum calcium and elevated alkaline phosphatase levels. Low Vitamin E would explain the hemolytic anemia. Low vitamin A levels would explain the conjunctiva injection which would be due to follicular conjunctivitis.

17) A) Given the history of a home delivery and no mention of the infant being given Vitamin K, the most likely explanation for the clinical manifestations would be hemorrhagic disease of the newborn due to factors, 2, 7, 9 and 10 deficiency.

The most appropriate treatment would be 2 units Vitamin K.

18) C) Both preterm and full term infants require 100-120 Kcal/ Kg /day to grow. In preterm infants this may be more difficult to achieve on standard formula which is why they require preterm formula which has more calories per ml.

19) B) The most common electrolyte abnormality during the first week of refeeding in a malnourished patient with anorexia nervosa is **hypo**phosphatemia. It is not clear what mechanism is responsible for that, but now you at least know what the correct answer would be if this pops up on the boards.

20) C) The most likely explanation for the patient's clinical presentation would be Galactose-1-phosphate uridyltransferase deficiency resulting in *galactosemia*. Infants with galactosemia are prone to gram negative sepsis such as E. coli. Hepatomegaly, elevated indirect bilirubin and positive reducing substances all go along with a diagnosis of galactosemia.

There is a risk for development of cataracts and they should be fed soy formula.

Preventive Pediatrics

21) D) Drowning deaths and injuries occur 4 times as often in boys. The surrounding fence is a critical component to preventing drowning, a concept frequently tested on the exam. Infant and toddler swimming lessons, while cute and enjoyable for parents, have not been proven to prevent drowning. Children in this age group lack the ability to understand safety issues; if anything, it gives a false sense of security.

In fact the AAP has a policy statement that swimming lessons should not be started prior to 4 years of age.

22) D) The most common agent for causing burns in children is hot liquid. This can occur either by immersion or via a spill. Spills occur primarily in children younger than 4 years.

23) B) A sibling who is older than 6, whose immunizations are up to date, and who has received the latest booster within 3 years would need no additional immunizations. However, prophylactic antibiotics are necessary for all household contacts and other close contacts such as those who attend daycare with the index case.

24) C) Each of the choices is a rare complication of the varicella vaccine except for temporal lobe seizures. In addition to the side effects listed, Guillain-Barré syndrome and Stevens-Johnson syndrome have been seen after administration of the varicella vaccine.

25) D) The varicella vaccine is contraindicated in all of these situations except HIV-positive children who are *asymptomatic* or *mildly symptomatic*.[2] At the present time there are protocols whereby children with ALL can receive the vaccine *if they are in remission.* Those not in remission cannot receive the vaccine.

26) A) "Egg-Xactly."[3] Substituting egg whites (notice we did not say egg yolk) for fat is a good way to reduce fat/cholesterol in the diet.

Nonfat and low-fat milks are not recommended for use during the first 2 years of life because of lower caloric density compared with whole-fat products. Total cholesterol or HDL does *not* require fasting but calculation of LDL *does.*

Regarding puberty, there is an increase in cholesterol levels just before puberty and a decrease during the growth spurt.

Poisons and Toxins

27) D) Administering activated charcoal at 0.5-1 Gram / Kg would be appropriate for the acute immediate management of ingestion of most pills including those that can be lethal in children. There are a few contraindications including heavy metals such as iron and metal salts such as lithium.

Ingestion of hydrocarbons including kerosene place a child at high risk for aspiration, which makes activated charcoal a contraindication. Cyanide is poorly absorbed by activated charcoal and therefore inactivate charcoal in the acute setting would be inappropriate.

Remember CALM, the substances charcoal is NOT a good choice for: cyanide, alcohol, lithium, and heavy metals. And, as listed above, it is not a good choice for hydrocarbons (gasoline, kerosene, lighter fluid, etc) or in many cases involving an antidote because it will absorb the antidote as well.

Activated charcoal would however be appropriate for suspected ingestion of beta blockers which is choice D.

28) D) The initial treatment for a child who likely ingested salicylates would include activated charcoal, and obtaining serum electrolytes as well as an acetaminophen level for possible co-ingestion. Once the electrolytes were obtained, calculating the anion gap would be important since the anion gap would likely be elevated.

Gastric lavage is no longer indicated for most ingestions because the risks outweigh the benefits. Its use is reserved for potential life-threatening ingestions that occurred within 60 minutes of being seen.

ANSWERS: Fetus and Newborn

29) C) Windshield wiper fluid, cooking fuel, perfumes, and antifreeze contain **methanol**, which is fatal when ingested if untreated. This is one of the few, if not the only time, when **administration of ethanol** would be appropriate.

When methanol is ingested, it gets broken down to formaldehyde by alcohol dehydrogenase. Formaldehyde is neurotoxic and can be fatal as well. Ethanol or ethyl alcohol competes with this enzyme preferentially and is broken down to acetaldehyde which is not toxic. It is of course administered IV in a controlled environment not served in shot glasses.

30) D) Button batteries measuring 20 mm or **larger** are associated with the most severe outcome. Lithium based batteries are **more toxic**. Once button batteries have leaked, tissue damage **can** worsen even after the battery is removed.

Button batteries that have passed into the stomach may be monitored with serial x-rays every 12 hours, but they must be monitored to make sure they continue to move down and out.

31) B) The diarrhea was described as being mild and the fact that she has been able to drink watered down sports drinks without vomiting points away from severe dehydration or electrolyte imbalance as the cause of the symptoms in the vignette.

This narrows down the choices to "some medication" given by the nanny. Simethicone helps alleviate abdominal pain caused by gas but would not likely cause any side effects even if given in excessive amounts. However, loperamide is used to treat diarrhea and if given too frequently or in too high a dose could cause some of the symptoms in the vignette. It is an opiate receptor agonist and could cause the miosis, mild hypotension, sedation and ataxia described in the vignette. As they say, know before you go ...to the bathroom

Fetus and Newborn

32) E) Developmental dysplasia of the hip is more common among Caucasian babies than African-American babies. It is more common among females and full-term babies, as well as in those with breech presentation.

33) D) Omphaloceles are indeed associated with several anomalies, including Beckwith-Wiedemann syndrome. Additional associated findings of Beckwith-Wiedemann syndrome include macroglossia, macrosomia, and hypoglycemia.

Failure of the umbilical ring to contract is associated with herniation of the umbilical cord. Folate-deficient diets during pregnancy have been linked to spinal cord defects, not omphalocele.

Gastroschisis is a similar defect. However, with gastroschisis there is no membranous covering, the defect tends to be smaller, and it is not associated with Beckwith-Wiedemann syndrome. .

In gastroschisis, the abdominal contents may protrude through any defect in the abdominal wall, but in omphaloceles they may only protrude through the umbilical opening.

34) D) Erythema toxicum is a common lesion in newborns. Diffuse pustules with an erythematous base characterize it. It would be distinguished from a *Staph* infection by the presence of eosinophils when the contents of the pustules are examined under the microscope.

Dry peeling skin is common in newborns, especially those who are post term. *Miliaria crystallina* are vesicles that are a result of the accumulation of sweat just below the skin surface due to sweat gland obstruction. It resolves on its own.

The *yellow papules* on the hard palate are *Epstein's pearls,* and these too are a common finding in newborns. This resolves in weeks.

On the other hand, a midline skin tag on the spine can be benign, but it can also be a marker for more serious defect involving the spinal canal. Therefore, radiological studies such as an MRI are indicated.

35) C) It is most important to avoid cold stress with its metabolic consequences. This is particularly important with a premature baby. Choice D can be done later on, once the infant has been stabilized and you have ingested a couple of Almond Joy® bars to wake yourself up. This is consistent with assessing airway first, since setting up optimal conditions for evaluating the newborn would be the first step en route to evaluating the airway.

ANSWERS: Fetus and Newborn

36) **E)** The most important factor in determining bonding of father and child is presence in the DR. It enhances closeness with the mother and also insures bonding with the baby in the initial hours after birth. Due to such modern equipment like DVR recorders, and HDTV in delivery rooms, fathers can now be present and see the opening kickoff or the opening schtickoff on the Dr. Phil show.

Age is one of the factors. However, adolescent males tend not to bond as well. An estimated 80% of fathers are present for their baby's delivery; including fathers who attend and record C-sections with their phones.[4]

37) **B)** The correct answer is B. Here is a case where, as noted in our main text, it is important to put numbers into words. In this case, since you already know the diagnosis, it makes sense to place the description "hypochloremic metabolic alkalosis" on your scratch pad as a reminder of the corresponding lab findings seen with pyloric stenosis. You could then at least begin eliminating choices with low bicarb and a high chloride. This is a lot easier than reasoning it all out. There is plenty of time for that after you are board certified and can afford to be "certified bored".

38) **D)** Pyloric stenosis, with its progressive projectile vomiting and loss of HCl in emesis, results in *hypo*chloremic alkalosis; it occurs primarily in male *first-born* babies; and there is usually a history on the *maternal* side.

It is always best to correct any metabolic abnormalities preoperatively, especially the alkalosis in order to reduce the risk for post-op apnea. I have known few pediatricians who have palpated the fabled olive and some pediatric surgeons who palpated the olive *and* the pimento, mostly at the bottom of a martini glass when they are at home post call.

39) **E)** Since the mother was treated for eclampsia, it is likely that she was treated with magnesium sulfate, resulting in hypermagnesemia in the newborn. Watch for the proper spelling: hyper-*manganesemia* would not be a factor.

After the use of $MgSO_4$ within 24 hours of delivery, one should watch the newborn for signs of magnesium toxicity, including neuromuscular and respiratory depression.

The mechanism to explain this is as follows: acetylcholine in the motor nerve terminals acts on the myocardium by slowing the SA node impulse formation and prolonging conduction time but this is way too boring and really should be in a well hidden footnote at the bottom of the page.

---

[4] I always wonder whom they are going to show this to. Guests that won't leave?

40) E) This is the classic presentation of "congenital torticollis", and early diagnosis and passive stretching is all that is needed. Proper management should result in significant correction within a few months. Otherwise, referral to orthopedics is needed to "set things straight".

If the infant were older, and one did not feel the mass in the SCM, one might also look for reflux as a potential cause of torticollis. Sandifer syndrome refers to the association of seizure-like posturing or torticollis as well as the presence of GERD. Often there is no vomiting with this, but it is quite amenable to anti-reflux medication and other precautions like positioning and thickened feeds.

41) C) The ABG is consistent with metabolic alkalosis and their mentioning the child's being on furosemide (Lasix®) is your clue. The fact that the child has BPD is not critical to the question. The question could have simply asked you to make a diagnosis based on the ABG alone. Lasix® results in metabolic alkalosis by decreasing chloride in the urine and increasing bicarb urine loss.

42) E) This is a description of pseudotumor cerebri, and too much vitamin A can cause it.

43) A) In total anomalous pulmonary venous connection, the pulmonary veins do not go back to the left side of the heart as they should. This is the underlying problem. Findings on x-ray include diffuse granular pattern due to increased pulmonary vascular markings. You might see the snowman sign or figure 8, but rarely before 4 months of age. This is due to cardiomegaly.

In early infancy you could see mild cyanosis, and signs of failure (dyspnea, tachypnea, tachycardia, and hepatomegaly).

There is no evidence of RDS or Group B Strep pneumonia. Cardiomegaly would not be a part of the clinical picture seen in transient tachypnea.

44) D) The clinical picture is a relatively benign one and is consistent with a diagnosis of transient tachypnea of the newborn which is self limited and improves with supportive care within a few hours.

ANSWERS: Fetus and Newborn

45) B) Approximately 10% of newborns require some form of resuscitation in the delivery room. This would include requiring tactile stimulation and oxygen and even some bag/mask ventilation.

46) E) Placing the baby on the mother to allow for breast feeding is important during the first hour when the baby is alert. Vitamin K, erythromycin, height and weight measurement can all wait for this, which should be given top priority even if the staff is due for their break in an hour.

47) C) Early discharge prior to 48 hours after a vaginal delivery and prior to 72 hours for C/section is an option if the infant is feeding well, stooled and voided and all screening tests are completed.

Early discharge is not okay if the mother is GBS positive.

48) D) The American Academy of Pediatrics recommends that all infants discharged prior to 72 hours be seen within 48 hours (2 days). This is assuming the absence of risk factors.

49) D) Breast feeding jaundice which might be described as *"breastfeeding associated jaundice"* is due to initial poor caloric intake until milk "comes in". The decreased caloric intake increases the entero-hepatic circulation resulting in indirect hyperbilirubinemia.

50) C) Your first clue here should be the age of the infant, which rules out all the normal benign causes of hyperbilirubinemia. Breast feeding jaundice is seen in the first few post natal days and the clay colored stools would not explain human milk associated jaundice or Gilbert syndrome.

The only diagnosis to explain the clay colored stools (acholic) is cholestasis.

51) D) *Conjugated hyperbilirubinemia* is defined as conjugated bilirubin greater than 2.0 or greater than 20% of the total bilirubin. Even though they are used interchangeably direct hyperbilirubinemia and conjugated hyperbilirubinemia are not considered the same. [5]

Unconjugated hyperbilirubinemia is more common than conjugated and Gilbert syndrome is associated with unconjugated hyperbilirubinemia.

Conjugated hyperbilirubinemia is not always associated with cholestasis. Rotor and Dubin Johnson syndromes are two examples that are not associated with cholestasis.

52) E) This is a typical presentation of a trachea-esophageal fistula (TE fistula), probably with a blind pouch esophagus connecting to the trachea. This is the most common variety of TE fistula, and it presents as choking episodes with feeding and the production of copious secretions. A feeding tube will appear coiled up in the blind pouch-ending esophagus on x-ray.

There is nothing in the history to suggest choanal atresia; therefore insertion of a catheter into both nares and/or a CT scan would not be indicated.

53) A) Fetal exposure to indomethacin increases risk for oligohydramnios, periventricular leukomalacia, and necrotizing enterocolitis (due to cerebral and splanchnic vasoconstriction). There is also a risk for *reversible* not *irreversible* renal failure.

54) C) Gastroesophageal reflux can present with chronic wheezing and, in severe cases, failure to thrive. Regurgitation typically occurs 30 minutes after a feeding, and irritability during or after feedings is a common finding.

However, the latest studies show that there is no proven beneficial effect of head elevation in the supine position.

---

[5] I doubt you will have to know why but if you are a glutton for punishment here goes, direct bilirubin may include both the conjugated fraction and bilirubin bound to albumin (delta bilirubin) and therefore …. Zzzzz. I think you get the picture.

ANSWERS: Fluids and Lytes

55) **E)** Rumination is the repeated and painless regurgitation of ingested food into the mouth. Usually it occurs soon after food is ingested. It is often seen in cases of neglect and there is a strong behavioral / psychological component.

Symptoms do not occur during sleep, and do not respond to standard treatment for gastroesophageal reflux. Symptoms must be present for 8 weeks or longer to establish a diagnosis.

Rumination is *not* associated with retching.

Fluids and Lytes

56) **A)** Some of you might have remembered something about a ratio of 3:1. However that will only get you as far as narrowing it down choices A and D.

The correct answer is 3:1 glucose: sodium. Glucose: sodium ratio *greater than* 3:1 results in an increased risk for osmotic diarrhea. Another important piece of information is the glucose content, which should be 2-2.5% with a sodium concentration of 60-90 mEq/L.

57) **D)** With **_acute_ hyponatremia** resulting in seizures, the goal is to *rapidly raise the serum sodium concentration by 3-6 mEq/L over a few minutes*. Remember it is 3% Saline NOT 0.3%. They have been known to play a number and decimal point shell game to trick you.

58) **C)** Hypernatremia results in the intracellular generation of idiogenic osmoles in brain tissue. This is to maintain homeostasis between intracellular and extracellular fluids. With correction it takes several hours for this to reverse and if the serum sodium concentration were to be changed too rapidly, fluid would rush in and cause cerebral edema and, subsequently, seizure.

59) E) This is a typical history and description of hypernatremic dehydration, especially the "doughy skin"; therefore, the serum sodium concentration of 165 mEq/L is the best answer.

60) B) *Hyperkalemia* is an associated electrolyte abnormality seen with HUS. The toxin impairs absorption of sodium by intestinal cells in villi leading to hyponatremia. In addition the toxin causes cell death, resulting in the movement of potassium from intracellular to extracellular space leading to hyperkalemia.

Endothelial cell injury is an important component of HUS, leading to platelet aggregation and consumptive thrombocytopenia.

Metabolic acidosis and hyperphosphatemia are also seen in HUS.

61) E) Metabolic owing to poor tissue oxygenation would be the only logical answer since the carbon dioxide is not in a range to result in acidosis secondary to CO_2 retention. Decreased pulmonary function at the small airway level results in poor oxygenation leading to lactic acid accumulation secondary to anaerobic respiration and resulting in **increased acidosis at the tissue level.** There is nothing to suggest a renal or cardiac cause. Excessive carbon dioxide loss would result in alkalosis, not acidosis as suggested by the pH of 7.25.

62) D) In the face of hypernatremia, idiogenic osmoles are produced by CNS tissue to maintain fluid volume. If hypernatremia is corrected too quickly for the idiogenic osmoles to fade away, it could result in cerebral edema.

CNS is the only tissue where idiogenic osmoles are produced. In most, but not all, cases the testes are not a part of the CNS.

63) B) Hypertension is frequently seen in Cushing syndrome. Edema is rarely seen. One would also expect so see increased body weight and serum sodium within normal range.

ANSWERS: Fluids and Lytes

64) D) Pneumonia, asthma, salicylate toxicity, and pulmonary edema can all result in respiratory alkalosis.

Barbiturate toxicity would result in respiratory *acidosis.*

65) D) Spinal cord injury, myasthenia crisis, Guillain-Barré syndrome and botulism are associated with acute neuromuscular disease and can cause respiratory acidosis.

Nicotine toxicity is more likely to cause respiratory *alkalosis.*

66) D) Hyperventilation and dyspnea are seen in severe acidemia. Arteriole dilation and insulin resistance are also seen in the face of severe acidemia.

Cardiac contractility is decreased not enhanced in severe acidemia.

67) D) Diarrhea, pancreatic fistula, hypoaldosteronism, and renal tubular acidosis are all causes of metabolic acidosis with a *normal anion gap.* Other causes are ureterostomy, small bowel fistula, extra chloride, and carbonic anhydrase inhibitor use.

Ethylene glycol toxicity is associated with a metabolic acidosis with an *elevated anion gap.*

Genetics

68) **B)** Down syndrome secondary to standard trisomy and Down syndrome due to translocation are phenotypically indistinguishable. While women older than 35 are at greater risk for having a child with Down syndrome, women in their 20s have more children with Down syndrome, simply because women in this age group have more babies. Had the question asked which age group has the higher "percentage" of babies with Down syndrome, clearly it would be women older than 35.

If the mother is carrying a translocation, the risk of recurrence is higher than if the father was the carrier. If neither parent is a carrier, the risk of recurrence is only 1%.

69) **B)** You may not know or care to know about the details of the sequence or even what the q27 is referring to. The reference to the X chromosome should make the question simpler than it appears. Keep in mind that on the general pediatric board exam they would not expect you to know esoteric references to something discussed in the darkest caverns of genetics meetings under candlelight.

All you need to know here is that you have a "male" patient diagnosed with intellectual disability and there is something "going on" with the X chromosome. That would tell you that the patient has fragile X syndrome. You could then rephrase the question to **"Which of the following are associated with fragile X syndrome?"** and then the answer is clearly macroorchidism, which is not a "big deal".

70) **A)** Since it is an "X-linked" recessive disorder, a male child who is unaffected does not have the genetic material. That is to say, there are no male carriers, and boys either have the disease or they don't and they are not carriers.

It is easy to get mislead and distracted into thinking the question is "additional children" in the existing family and not about future grandchildren. If you did not read the question carefully you would have found yourself "swimming with the red herrings".

ANSWERS: Genetics

71) A) Children with Cri-du –Chat syndrome present with epicanthal folds, cardiac defects, psychomotor retardation and *micro*cephaly. They do not present with *macro*cephaly.

72) D) Russel Silver syndrome is associated with cardiac defects, abnormalities in the 5th finger, triangle face with normal head circumference. However wide spaced teeth are not part of the syndrome.

73) C) The description is classic of Cornelia de Lange Syndrome.

74) E) Macroglossia, hemihypertrophy, cardiomegaly, and hepatomegaly are all consistent with a diagnosis of Beckwith-Wiedemann syndrome.

75) C) The broad thumb and great toe should be enough information to make the diagnosis. Throw in the beaked nose and cardiac abnormalities and answering this one correctly should be a piece of cake.

76) C) The karyotype most associated with Klinefelter syndrome is XXY not XYY and it is the leading cause of male infertility. Males with Klinefelter syndrome are at increased risk for developing breast cancer. While children with Klinefelter have normal intellectual ability, it is considered to be *slightly decreased* compared to the rest of the population.

Testosterone replacement is part of the treatment. Other features of Klinefelter syndrome include tall stature with long arms and leg, mildly delayed motor and language development, and a "calm demeanor". They may be described as being shy and sedentary.

77) B) Valproic acid can result in neural tube defects, short palpebral fissures, short nose, and straight contour to the upper vermillion border, cardiac defects, and mental retardation

ACE inhibitors can impact renal development negatively. Warfarin can lead to marked nasal hypoplasia and stippling of the epiphyses. Carbamazepine use, especially during the first trimester, increases the risk for neural tube defects, small short nose and small fingernails.

Heparin is considered to be safe during pregnancy.

An important fact to keep in mind is that fetal alcohol syndrome has physical features that overlap with exposure to anticonvulsants however fetal alcohol syndrome also results in babies being SGA and microcephalic.

78) D) The features described are a result of malformation as a result of mechanical forces which one would expect with oligohydramnios.

None of the other choices could explain the described features.

79) D) TEF is considered to be a "multifactorial trait". Since this cannot be traced to a single gene the specific genetic pattern cannot be identified. However there is an increased chance of conceiving a 2nd child with the defect than in the general population. The risk for conceiving another child with the same defect is 4%.

Single malformations due to a multifactorial inheritance pattern are the most common type of major anomaly seen. Other examples include pyloric stenosis, Hirschsprung disease, cleft lip with cleft palate, cleft lip and spina bifida.

80) E) Exposure to ACE inhibitors would best explain the findings of patent ductus arteriosis and fetal anuria.

81) D) The combination of thyroid disturbance and atrial septal defect would be consistent with fetal exposure to lithium. In addition infants exposed to lithium are at risk for Ebstein anomaly.

Allergy and Immunology

82) 1) C
      2) D
      3) A
      4) B

      An Arthus/ Immune complex reaction is a Type 3 allergic reaction

      A delayed hypersensitivity reaction such as contact dermatitis is a Type 4 reaction

      An anaphylactoid reaction would be a Type 1 allergic reaction

      A Type 2 allergic reaction is antibody mediated

83) D) Common variable immunodeficiency can result in both defects in cell mediated immunity and hypoglobulinemia. Patients will present with recurrent respiratory problems and occasionally vague GI symptoms and anemia. A poor response to the vaccine wouldn't explain the recurrent respiratory symptoms. X-linked severe immunodeficiency would have a much more (as the name implies) severe picture and HIV would not likely present with a thriving child with a negative physical examination, especially on the Boards.

84) E) Since they note that the baby is being exclusively breast fed, the rash is probably related to this. The description is of atopic dermatitis. It is very possible that something in the mother's diet is responsible and the allergen is crossing over into the breast milk, causing a reaction in the infant. Skin testing the mother will not be of help since she is not the one with the rash.

Skin testing the infant will not be helpful due to the fact that the rash is diffuse and the infant has been given diphenhydramine.

The antihistamine will interfere with the accuracy of the skin testing. The presence of IgE in the infant to various allergens will help determine the cause. Switching to soy formula may not be of help since the infant may have been sensitized to soy formula as well.

85) C) IgA deficiency is the most common primary immunodeficiency. Since this is the antibody found in mucosal linings, it results in frequent infections of the respiratory, GI, and urogenital tracts.

86) E) Thymic transplantation is most successful in patients with complete DiGeorge syndrome who have a significant T-lymphocyte deficiency.

87) E) B cells in patients with x-linked hyper IgM syndrome can make IgM but cannot make IgG, IgA or IgE. Therefore IgM levels are high and IgG, IgA, and IgE levels are low.

Treatment with intravenous gammaglobulin is indicated. In addition these patients are at increased risk for infection with P. jiroveci and prophylaxis is indicated.

88) D) IgA deficiency is the *most* common primary immunodeficiency. Most patients with this disorder are actually asymptomatic.

Symptomatic cases usually also have defects in one or more IgG subclasses.

IgA deficiency is *not* an indication for replacement immunoglobulin therapy.

Patients with IgA deficiency often have circulating anti-IgA antibody. Even though most commercial IgG preparations contain negligible amounts of IgA, even this small amount can cause an anaphylactoid reaction in patients with IgA deficiency.

89) C) Growth velocity is reduced during the first year of treatment. However catchup growth after the first year results in the achievement of adult height.

Inhaled steroids are not risk-free. Acne, mood swings and weight gain do occur although not as frequently as is seen with systemic steroid use.

Oral candidiasis is one of the more common complications but is reduced with mouth-rinsing after inhalation.

ANSWERS: Infectious Disease

90) E) Topical diphenhydramine would likely irritate the skin and topical hydrocortisone would have no long term role intreating chronic urticaria

Hydroxyzine and diphenhydramine can be sedating making them poor candidates for long term treatment.

Fexofenadine is a 2nd generation non sedating H1 antihistamine and would be the most appropriate long term treatment for chronic urticaria of those listed.

Infectious Disease

91) C) **The 3 C's of measles are cough, coryza, and conjunctivitis** Patients are contagious from 2 days before becoming symptomatic until 4 days after the onset of the rash.

While hand washing is a good idea with any infectious disease, measles is spread by droplets of respiratory secretions so **isolation** is the key to preventing the spread of disease not hand washing.

Encephalitis is not a common complication; it is a rare complication, affecting 1:1000 cases, and is insidious in onset not acute in onset. Subacute sclerosing panencephalitis occurs up to a decade later.

Measles specific IgM levels would be helpful if obtained **2 weeks later**, not at presentation. In addition, it is important to always consider measles when you see the word *coryza* in the history.

92) E) Pregnant women should not receive this live vaccine. However, children who are HIV positive and asymptomatic with high CD4 value should receive the vaccine because the benefits outweigh the risks. HIV patients with low CD4 values should not receive the MMR vaccine because vaccine related pneumonia have been reported.

A symptomatic HIV patient should receive IG prophylaxis regardless of immunizations status

Any individual born before 1957 would likely be immune. The vaccine would be helpful only if given within **3-days (72 hour) of exposure**. A child who is younger than 12 months might not develop a strong enough immune response and should therefore receive immunoglobulin. They would also still need TWO more measles vaccines after age 12 months; the one received before that would not be counted.

93) A) Rubella is actually a very mild disease. **In fact, routine vaccination is really to prevent disease in pregnant women and is the only vaccine given to provide protection for someone other than the child on the receiving end of the needle.** It is so mild that in the pre vaccine era, the disease was often inapparent.

The period of communicability begins 2 days before the appearance of the rash and lasts another 7 days. Infants with congenital rubella are considered contagious through body secretions up to *1 year after birth.* Therefore E "could be true" so it is not the correct choice and besides I threw in the Oktoberfest line to remind you that rubella is also known as German measles, but Rubella is the term they will toss around on the Boards.

94) E) Remember the **RIP** mnemonic. Confirmed cases of tuberculosis consists of treatment with **r**ifampin, **i**soniazid and **p**yrazinamide.

95) E) Administration with BCG can result in a false positive result not a false negative result. All of the other choices can result in a false negative.

96) C) The rapidity of onset and intensity of local pain, swelling, and erythema are characteristic of *Pasteurella multocida* infection. This organism is associated with up to 80% of cat bite infections and is found in the mouths of approximately 65% of cats. *P. multocida* would likely be resistant to penicillin, making it an inappropriate choice. First-generation cephalosporins have limited activity against this organism. Amoxicillin/clavulanic acid would be effective against *Pasteurella multocida.* Clindamycin and Septra would be appropriate for penicillin allergic patients.

97) B) Herpes simplex virus grows readily in cell culture, and special transport media are available for specimens that cannot be inoculated immediately. Serologic tests generally are not helpful for the diagnosis of acute HSV infection. Viral culture would be the most specific diagnostic test.

ANSWERS: Infectious Disease

98) B) With community acquired MRSA becoming more pervasive, the most appropriate initial treatment in this setting would be trimethoprim with sulfamethoxazole, or clindamycin, depending on local resistance.

99) E) Despite the findings consistent with otitis media, a full sepsis workup including lumbar puncture is indicated. Therefore, PO amoxicillin would not be appropriate. In this age group you must provide coverage for group B *Strep, Pneumococcus, Meningococcus,* and *Listeria* monocytogenes. IV ampicillin for *Listeria* and gentamicin for the other bugs would provide appropriate initial coverage until a bacterial infection has been ruled out or an organism identified.

In addition ampicillin and gentamicin would have a synergistic effect against Listeria.

100) E) Whenever you see the combination of
- renal problems
- anemia,
- thrombocytopenia,

You should automatically think of hemolytic uremic syndrome (HUS). This often manifests with fragmented RBCs and a high BUN and creatinine.

Young children are at greatest risk when exposed to the etiological agent.[6] It occurs after exposure to contaminated food, typically undercooked meat, although it can be contracted from dairy products and vegetables as well. Antibiotics are **not** routinely indicated nor are agents that stop the diarrhea. These can both make the situation worse.

101) B) The clinical scenario presented, staccato cough, diffuse infiltrates, and increased eosinophilia in an afebrile infant of this age, is most likely *Chlamydia trachomatis*. PO erythromycin would be the most appropriate treatment.

102) B) Azithromycin would be indicated for all household contacts as well as other close contacts *regardless of immunization status.*

Erythromycin is for preventing the further spread of infection.

---

[6] *E. Coli* 0157:H7 for those into such details.

103) B) Aminoglycosides such as gentamicin can result in blockade at the neuromuscular junction. Therefore, they should be avoided in patients with underlying neuromuscular disorders.

104) D) CMV, adenovirus, Human herpes virus (HHV)-6 and rubella can present with a clinical picture similar to EBV infectious mononucleosis.

Paramyxovirus, does not present with such a clinical picture.

In particular, CMV can also include atypical lymphs on the CBC. Look for hints in the question that EBV is the incorrect answer and CMV is the correct choice.

105) D) Discarding the box when it is full is the rule of thumb. When it comes to recapping needles, one hand is better than two because of the increased risk of missing and getting stuck.[7] When they work right,[8] retractable needles are the better option. Needles and sharps should never be passed to another person, and the sharp container should be accessible to health care staff but not patients, especially pediatric patients.

106) B) This is an example where reading the question is critical. The question asked for the most common "cutaneous" manifestation, while condylomata lata is *a* manifestation of secondary syphilis, not a "cutaneous" manifestation. Condylomata lata are gray-white wartlike lesions found on mucous membrane tissues.

107) A) Among the choices given, CMV is the only correct one. Somewhere in the recesses of your board preparing cluttered mind you say you recall that rubeola also can result in deafness. Well, if rubeola "rings a bell" it is because sensorineural deafness can occur with congenital ru*bella* infection. It is very easy to avoid confusion in the future if you picture the "bell" in rubella ringing loud enough to cause deafness and loud enough to get the correct answer on the exam. In other words, when you see rubella as one of the choices a "little bell" should go off in your head. Rubeola should not.

---

[7] Just think of the paperwork alone.
[8] When is that?

ANSWERS: Infectious Disease

108) **D)** You may have remembered Fitz Hugh Curtis, but it is also important to remember that this is *perihepatitis* and not hepatitis. The combination of joint symptoms coupled with right upper quadrant pain should help you identify gonorrhea as the correct answer.

Fitz Hugh Curtis may be a manifestation of chlamydia infection as well.

109) **D)** Whenever a "park cleanup" is involved, "bird droppings" should be considered a prime suspect in the etiology of the presenting symptoms. In such cases you are down to two choices, cryptococcosis and histoplasmosis. With cryptococcosis, they will often describe and/or emphasize a headache.

Histoplasmosis is found throughout the Ohio, Missouri and Mississippi river valleys. Hepatosplenomegaly helps differentiate it from the other flu-like illnesses. Treatment is supportive for immunocompetent children, while immunocompromised children with disseminated disease require Amphotericin B.

110) **B)** An infant with lesions on the palms and soles along with hepatosplenomegaly would most likely have congenital syphilis. Another classic gift they might hand you is "snuffles" or copious nasal secretions. The decreased movement of the extremities is known as "pseudoparalysis" and the anemia is a "hemolytic" anemia.

111) **C)** If you are presented with a school aged child with clinical signs of pneumonia, especially with fever and malaise with a chest x-ray demonstrating bilateral diffuse infiltrates, you should consider a diagnosis of mycoplasma pneumonia.

The best treatment for mycoplasma would be azithromycin.

112) **C)** You would need to cover for beta lactamase producing organisms including non typeable H. flu and M. catarrhalis. Using even higher dose amoxicillin won't help since they already noted that high dose amoxicillin was used. Azithromycin will not be effective against beta lactamase producing organisms.

Cipro and tetracycline would not be appropriate in a 7 year old and the argument stops there.

113) A) Clindamycin, Trimethoprim/sulfamethoxazole, linezolid and vancomycin are all appropriate choices for the initial treatment of methicillin resistant Staph aureus infections. Amoxicillin/clavulanic acid would not since these organisms are not sensitive to it.

114) B) Rifampin is the mainstay prophylaxis for exposure to meningococcal sepsis. Any healthcare worker who examined the patient's throat or intubated the patient would be considered to be a close contact in need of prophylaxis. The appropriate dose for an adult would be 600 mg BID for 2 days. The maximum dose is 600 mg therefore 1200 mg q day for 4 days would be incorrect.

Ceftriaxone 250 mg IM would be okay but who would want a shot when one dose of ciprofloxacin can be given. It was important that the question stated that this is a male resident. Had it been a female resident the possibility of pregnancy would exist and ciprofloxacin would be inappropriate.

The meningococcal vaccine can be given as an adjunctive treatment in addition to antibiotics if it is due to a susceptible strain. Serotype A is a susceptible strain.

A, C, Y and W-135[9] are all susceptible strains (might be easier to remember as YWCA especially if you picture women Village People dancing), and now there is a new vaccine for strain B.

115) C) The most common mode of transmission is via contaminated food. Mothers of affected infants are usually symptomatic with flulike symptoms a few days prior to delivery. However, there is a later onset form of listeriosis where the mothers are asymptomatic. However in early onset disease, which is the more common form, mothers are usually asymptomatic.

Contrary to the species name "monocytogenes", there is no monocytosis associated with listeriosis nor is there monocytopenia or leukopenia. However leukocytosis is an associated finding.

116) C) Listeria is always resistant to cephalosporins and therefore cefotaxime and ceftriaxone would be inappropriate. Ampicillin would of course be inappropriate in a penicillin allergic patient.

Chloramphenicol has a high failure rate and has side effects that would make it inappropriate. Trimethoprim –sulfamethoxazole is bacteriocidal and reaches good levels in the CSF.

---

[9] Why are they called, A, C , Y and W-135? Do you care? Just remember these are the susceptible strains!

ANSWERS: Infectious Disease

117) E) In a routine case of CSD in an immunocompetent patient the appropriate treatment is nothing more than supportive care. Lymph node biopsy would be reserved for atypical cases and cases where diagnosis cannot be confirmed by any other means.

118) A) Incubation periods are *shorter* in children. Patients on chronic steroids, or who sustain bites closer to the CNS and/or multiple bites can expect a shorter incubation period. The mean incubation is 30-90 days.

119) D) While one could argue that A "Beam me up Scotty I have one for Mr. Spock" is correct it would not be the best answer, although very logical. You would have to read the question and more importantly write down what each serum marker means in words.

For example:
HBsAb = Hepatitis B Surface antibody
HBsAg = Hepatitis B Surface antigen
HBcAb = Hepatitis B core antibody

This makes it much easier to interpret with Spock-like rational interpretation devoid of any emotion.

In this case, the HBsAb and HBcAb are negative. Therefore any choices referencing immunity are logically incorrect.

Since the HBsAg is positive, you are dealing with an active infection.

120) B) While one could argue that choice E is correct which spells out "Help, my eyes are so glazed over moths have been landing on my eyes without my noticing" would be correct it shouldn't, if you just follow the moth to the light.

If you are asked a question regarding the "replication rate" or "infectivity" of hepatitis B, then you are dealing with the e antigen.

So now that you see the light, hopefully the moths will follow suit and leave your eyes and head to the light themselves.

121) C) While one could argue that choice E is correct which spells out

"How the heck should I know" is the correct answer? However, you really should know as follows:

Remember, antibodies imply immunity, so look for something with an "Ab" positive. HbsAb would be positive with either immunity from vaccination or from natural disease.

If the HBcAb is positive, however, this means the immunity is from natural disease..

Now you should be asking "HowtheheckcanIgetthiswrong?" = "How the heck can I get this wrong"?

Inborn Errors of Metabolism

122) A) Hunter's syndrome is X-linked recessive. This is best remembered by envisioning hunters using X's at the end of their bows and arrows when they hunt. In addition most hunters are male and X-linked recessive disorders affect males.

123) 1) C
2) B
3) B
4) A
5) D

Both Hurlers and Hunters syndromes present with coarse facies. Only Hurlers presents with corneal clouding after all, you can't see if you are a hunter and have corneal clouding!

Hunter's syndrome is X-linked recessive. Skeletal involvement and normal intelligence would describe Morquio syndrome which is not included in this question.

124) E) Phenylketonuria (PKU) is the most plausible explanation for the situation described in the question. In the real world it would be unusual for a patient to present at 6 months due to diligent screening required by law. However, this is the Boards, a world unto itself. It is recommended that the blood for screening be obtained after 48–72 hours of life and preferably after feeding proteins in order to reduce the possibility of false-negative results.

ANSWERS: Inborn Errors of Metabolism

125) B) Ornithine transcarbamoylase deficiency is a urea cycle defect and therefore would indeed be associated with elevated serum ammonia levels. Elevated serum ammonia levels are also seen in methylmalonic acidemia.

Reye's syndrome and other diseases associated with liver failure result in elevated serum ammonia levels.

Like Reye's syndrome, Leigh disease is also associated with encephalopathy; however, it is not associated with elevated serum ammonia levels.

126) E) The vignette describes **Lesch Nyhan syndrome**, which is categorized by self-mutilation. Because of the abnormal movements, it can be confused with athetoid cerebral palsy. However, the choices point to a specific metabolic disorder and the typical features of Lesch Nyhan are being described. Please note that uric acid levels are for diagnostic purposes only. Bringing the uric acid levels under control will *not* help control any of the neurological or behavioral manifestations of the disorder.

127) A) The combination of physical and lab findings makes for a diagnosis of Von Gierke disease which is glycogen storage disease type 1 (GSD 1).

GSD I is due to glucose 6-phophatase deficiency which impedes the breakdown of glycogen into glucose.

This results in the **accumulation of glucose -6-phosphate. which leads to increased lactic acid**

Hepatomegaly results along with failure to thrive.

Elevated uric acid levels, ketonuria hyperlipidemia also result. Clinically seizures are also a common presentation.

Treatment is the frequent feeding of carbohydrates such as corn starch.

Pompe Disease is also known as GSD type 2 and it is due to a deficiency in the lysosomal breakdown of glycogen. Presentation is also of a hypotonic nonthriving infant in the first month of life, but these infants may have cardiomegaly and "hard muscles" and fascinatingly, NO hypoglycemia.

128) E) Most infants identified in newborn screening with elevated phenylalanine (PA) levels won't have PKU. In some cases it might be due to delayed maturation of metabolizing enzymes. Others might have biopterin deficiency.

The bottom line is infants identified in PKU screening require additional workup before concluding that they have PKU.

129) D) The patient's newborn screening and anterior fontanelle make hypothyroid unlikely. There is nothing to suggest myasthenia gravis, mitochondrial disorder or glycogen storage disorder, making for a most likely diagnosis of botulism poisoning. The introduction of cereal was mentioned for a reason. Honey might have been part of the preparation.

130) D) The combination of hemolysis, liver disease with preceding neurological signs makes for a diagnosis of Wilson disease and thus a serum ceruloplasmin would be the most helpful test.

Endocrinology

131) B) In most states, the newborn screen for hypothyroidism measures TSH levels. A positive screen needs to be confirmed by measuring a serum TSH and free T4 levels. However treatment should be started before the results are confirmed.

132) E) Children who develop hypothyroidism after 3 years of age won't develop *permanent* impairment of intellectual or neurological function. In this case it is important to read the question carefully. There can be impairment but it is reversible with treatment, therefore the italicized word *permanent* is important here.

ANSWERS: Endocrinology

133) C) The most appropriate treatment for idiopathic central precocious puberty is leuprolide which is GnRH agonist. This works by down regulating the GnRH and suspending premature pubertal development.

134) C) The combination of a drop-off in height, maintenance of weight and pubertal delay points to hypothyroidism, Cushing disease or growth hormone deficiency.

With familial short stature one would expect to see low percentile for height and weight maintained from birth to adulthood. In constitutional growth delay one would expect bone age below chronological age however one would not expect a drop-off in the height curve.

In Crohn disease and nutritional deficiency one would not expect to see maintenance of weight in the 50th percentile.

Their mentioning that the other sibling was a slow grower is a red herring.

135) D) Erythrocyte sedimentation rate

The combination of drop-off in both weight and height points to a gastrointestinal disorder such as Crohn disease. Therefore of the choices listed the most appropriate initial screen would be an erythrocyte sedimentation rate.

136) D) Of the choices listed the best screen for growth hormone deficiency would be IGF-1 which stands for "Insulin like growth factor – 1". Another correct choice if it were listed is "Insulin like growth factor binding protein – 3".

137) D) If you suspect a diagnosis of celiac disease in a child and have documented normal IgA concentrations the most appropriate initial screen would be tissue transglutaminase antibody level.

138) D) The history is consistent with delayed puberty due to a central nervous system cause most likely a pituitary tumor. Of all the choices the most appropriate study to order would be a serum prolactin level which would be elevated with a pituitary tumor. [10]

139) A) If you simply divide the parents' height in inches by 12 you discover that they are both around 5 feet tall. Clearly this boy will not be playing center in the NBA all-star game. Thus, the diagnosis is genetic short stature and "normal". The only pattern that makes sense, therefore, would be choice A.

140) E) The combination or normal Vitamin D 1, 25, Vitamin D, 25, serum calcium and parathyroid hormone along with elevated alkaline phosphatase and low serum phosphate in a child with clinical rickets is consistent with a diagnosis of familial hypophosphatemic rickets.

141) A) By noting that the infant is African American and lactose intolerant they are steering you toward a diagnosis of Vitamin D deficient rickets. There are two risk factors at play here. One risk factor is dark skin resulting in decreased exposure to ultraviolet light. Another is lactose intolerance which could result in decreased dairy product and Vitamin D intake.

The elevated PTH and alkaline phosphatase coupled with the decreased calcium, phosphate and 25-Vitamin D, confirms the correct diagnosis.

Hypophosphatasia is an inherited disorder of poor alkaline phosphatase production and not consistent with the clinical scenario in the question.

142) B) Vitamin D dependent rickets Type 1 is due to impaired production of Vitamin D 1, 25 by the kidney. This results in very low levels of Vitamin D1, 25 and no improvement with Vitamin D replacement as one would expect with Vitamin D deficient rickets.

---

[10] If you must know why this is because of pressure on the pituitary stalk resulting in disruption of dopaminergic inhibition of prolactin. Elevated prolactin levels would interfere with normal menstrual cycles and pubertal development. Now get back to work on material you might actually be tested on!

ANSWERS: Endocrinology

143) C) Hereditary Vitamin D Resistant Rickets (formerly known as Vitamin D Dependent Rickets Type 2) is due to end organ resistance to Vitamin D. Therefore the primary way to differentiate Type 1 from this is the Vitamin D 1, 25 levels which are very elevated in the resistant form and low in the dependent form.

144) B) Metabolic syndrome has some overlap with type 2 diabetes but it is not the same. There is some overlap but it is a different entity. However the important points to know are:

The International Diabetes foundation established the following criteria:

- Fasting triglycerides greater than 150
- High density lipoprotein cholesterol **less than** 40
- Blood pressure greater than 130/85
- Fasting glucose greater than 100 OR previously diagnosed with diabetes type 2

Acanthosis nigricans seen in diabetes type 2 is not a criterion for metabolic syndrome and neither is family history of diabetes type 2 disease.

145) E) When presented with unexplained deterioration or recurrent deterioration of a chronic condition in an adolescent, *poor compliance* should always be a consideration. This is the most likely explanation for the recurrent episodes of DKA in this otherwise appropriately managed teenager. The question notes that the patient is "on an appropriate insulin regimen" and the nutritionist has "set up" an appropriate diet. This does not mean the patient is compliant. If the patient was compliant this would have been specifically stated. Once again read the question carefully.

The Somogyi effect is is caused by nighttime hypoglycemia, which leads to a rebound hyperglycemia in the early morning hours.

The Dawn effect also presents as morning hyperglycemia. However it is not related to nocturnal hypoglycemia.

146) E) The younger the child is at the age of onset, the more likely they have Type 1 diabetes. Type 1 diabetes, in addition to being an autoimmune phenomenon, can also be "idiopathic".[11]

Type 2 is due to insulin resistance and some secretory deficits. While Type 2 disease is seen 'primarily' in obese children, if you assume a lean child cannot have Type 2 disease, you may misdiagnose and incorrectly manage the child.

147) 1) (B)
      2) (B)
      3) (B)
      4) (A)
      5) (C)
      6) (D)

An *incidental diagnosis* of Type 2 disease is in an otherwise asymptomatic patient is common. On the other hand Type 1 usually presents with notable symptoms. Type 2 can present with a vaginal monilial infection. Acanthosis nigricans is a hyperpigmentation noted in the skin folds of the neck and flexion areas. It is associated with insulin resistance.

One would only expect to see autoantibodies in Type 1 disease. Stress can exacerbate both Type 1 and Type 2 disease.

Arcaneis testus is Latin (or maybe Greek) for "arcane test", which is what the board exam is. It is believed that the recently retired system utilizing number two pencils and dots was actually used by Hippocrates when he "sat" for the boards.[12]

148) C) With the exception of the occasional red herring, there is a reason you are given each bit of information, including **the fact that the mother is a Type 1 diabetic. They do not mention that the child is diabetic and this is important** Type 1 diabetes is not known to have a genetic link, so any disturbance in glucose metabolism is probably not biological.

The source of the insulin is either endogenous or exogenous (i.e., in the cases involving Münchhausen by proxy). *The C-peptide levels correlate with the endogenously produced insulin. A high insulin level combined with a low C-peptide level indicates factitious hypoglycemia* and would implicate the mother. Nice work Dr. Gregory House! This would prove that the mother is administering exogenous insulin to the child, resulting in episodes of hypoglycemia and confirming a diagnosis of Münchhausen by proxy.

---

[11] Which is Latin for "We have no idea?"
[12] He also served as his own proctor the second time he took the exam.

ANSWERS: GI

149)
1) (C)
2) (B)
3) (C)
4) (D)
5) (D)
6) (B)
7) (B)

Hashimoto's thyroiditis is also known as chronic lymphocytic thyroiditis and can result in *hyper*thyroidism (hashitoxicosis) or *hypo*thyroidism. Both Graves' and Hashimoto's are triggered by components of the immune system: Hashimoto's by lymphocytic infiltration and Graves' by human thyroid stimulating hormone (which is an IgG). Neither one represents precancerous lesions. The owner of the diner on *Happy Days* was Arnold and, although he is of Japanese ancestry (and later starred in *The Karate Kid*); the actor is Noriyuki "Pat" Morita, not Hashimoto.

Patients with Hashimoto's disease can be clinically euthyroid or hypothyroid. Most are **asymptomatic** and are discovered by the presence of a goiter. In such cases T4 and TSH should be checked regularly.

GI

150) D) A low fat diet can contribute to non-specific diarrhea and therefore one of the steps in managing this condition is to increase fat in the diet. Therefore 2% milk could be a contributing factor. Switching to whole milk would be one way to manage help resolve the problem. Excessive bile acids can contribute and juices that have fructose concentrations *in excess* of glucose can also contribute to the condition.

151) B) Cholestyramine would be indicated if green stools were a part of the clinical picture; these would serve to bind fecal bile acids, a contributing factor in this form of diarrhea. Grape juice and orange juice contain fructose and glucose in a 1:1 ratio, which makes for better absorption of both. In addition, they contain no sorbitol, a major contributing factor to chronic non-specific diarrhea. On the other hand, pear and apple juice have high fructose to glucose ratios AND sorbitol, a double whammy. Fat intake and dietary fiber should both be **increased**, not decreased.

152) 1) B
2) C
3) D
4) A

An elevated ESR would correspond to the presence of chronic inflammation. Pernicious anemia could be seen on a routine CBC as macrocytic anemia.

Abnormalities of carbohydrate absorption could be assessed by measuring stool pH.

Disorders caused by disruption of the integrity of the intestinal lymphatic system could be diagnosed with a D-xylose absorption study.

153) C) The combination of bilious vomiting on all initial feedings along with a non-distended abdomen would suggest an upper GI obstruction distal to the pylorus. The double bubble sign would correspond with duodenal atresia and is the most likely diagnostic finding.

154) B) Irritable bowel syndrome is often precipitated by stress, resulting in recurrent diarrhea as well as crampy abdominal pain. Short stature is not part of the picture. While the presence of mucus in the stool is typical, hematochezia is not.

155) C) Indeed, here one has to read the question carefully. One would expect to find a sausage-like mass on the *right upper quadrant,* not the left lower quadrant. Bloody stools may not present until the first 12 hours, and this child became symptomatic 6 hours ago. Bilious vomiting can develop in patients with intussusception, and it is the most common cause of intestinal obstruction in children of age 3 months to 6 years.

Treatment of choice is air contrast enema, which is both diagnostic and therapeutic. Recurrence can occur 10% of the time, which means it does not in 90% of cases.

ANSWERS: GI

156) **A)** Ariboflavinosis is the deficiency of riboflavin. **Riboflavin's other name is vitamin B$_2$.** Ariboflavinosis is associated with **photophobia, blurred vision, burning** and **itching of the eyes, corneal vascularization, poor growth,** and <u>*cheilosis,*</u> which are cracks and sores on the outside of the lips. Xerophthalmia is excessive dryness of the cornea and conjunctiva, caused by a deficiency of vitamin A.

157) **C)** The explanation should simply state that recurrent diarrhea in this clinical setting is most suggestive of *Giardia lamblia.*

158) **E)** One would expect a patient to be low in albumin if they either:

Cannot produce it: End-stage liver disease

Cannot take it in: Kwashiorkor or other forms of malnutrition. *Intestinal lymphangiectasia* resulting in obstruction of intestinal vessels would also impact absorption

Lose it in the urine: Nephrotic syndrome

Lose it in the stool: Inflammatory bowel disease, protein losing enteropathies, celiac disease, or GI infectious diseases

However, hepatitis A would not result in end-stage liver disease nor would it result in hypoalbuminemia.

159) **B)** This would be consistent with a history of *Gilbert's disease*, which is an *autosomal dominant* disorder seen primarily in males. It is a benign disorder whose primary manifestation is a mild elevation of unconjugated bilirubin during times of high stress, such as physical training. One way to remember this is to think of a male named "Bert" with "gills" that gather in yellow dye, making him look yellow. This will help you remember that it affects males, the name Gilbert, and that it results in yellow color.

160) A) A *younger age of onset* represents a higher risk potential for developing hemolytic uremic syndrome after infection with enterohemorrhagic *E. coli*. Antimotility meds[13] should not be used since they can increase risk for hemolytic uremic syndrome in the face (no pun intended) of diarrhea.

Antibiotics can result in the increased release of the "vero toxin" when the *E. coli* cells are lysed.[14] Indeed, some studies have even suggested that toxin *production* could be increased. So, although not proven to worsen the prognosis, antibiotics are usually discouraged.

Elevated WBC and prolonged disease are both poor prognostic signs as well.

161) C) The key here is the recent use of amoxicillin. They could have mentioned the recent use of any antibiotic, which can lead to *pseudomembranous colitis.* This is where writing notes in the margins comes in handy. Remember, the disease can occur weeks after antibiotics have been discontinued. A toxin produced by *Clostridium difficile* is responsible.

Treatment involves stopping any antibiotics the patient is currently taking and starting oral metronidazole. *This is now the drug of choice to reduce the incidence of vancomycin-resistant Enterococci.*

Vancomycin would be used if there were *no response to metronidazole.* In addition, no treatment is needed initially if the patient is currently on antibiotics and the symptoms stop after the antibiotics are discontinued.

162) D) Alpha 1 antitrypsin deficiency is the most common genetic cause of both chronic and acute liver disease in children. It is also the most common genetically caused disorder requiring liver transplantation in children. It can present as neonatal hepatitis syndrome in children.

Mild elevation of transaminase values can be seen in toddlers.

163) D) Since this infant is asymptomatic other than intermittent emesis and is growing well all that is necessary is reassurance

It is always more appropriate to have the infant sleep in the supine position to reduce the risk of SIDS. Thickening formula or medications would not be appropriate in this setting

---

[13] Also known in some parts as the chemical plug.
[14] The toxin largely responsible for the syndrome.

ANSWERS: Pulmonary

164) E) Non-bilious vomiting is typically seen in rotavirus infection. Rotavirus is typically seen during the winter months and often can include respiratory symptoms.

If you are presented with a child with bloody diarrhea, a diagnosis of rotavirus gastroenteritis will lead you down the primrose path of an incorrect answer.

165) B) There are two currently licensed Rotavirus vaccines. The 1st dose should not be given later than 12 weeks of age and the 3rd dose no later than 32 weeks of age.

The risk for intussusception for the most recently licensed vaccines was similar for placebo.

Pulmonary

166) D) Bronchiectasis is a *permanent* dilation of bronchi or bronchioles in a particular segment of lung, resulting in recurrent infections involving the same lung segment. Symptoms often increase when the patient is lying down. It is best diagnosed by CT scan.

167) A) The best explanation would be persistent hypoventilation following hyaline membrane disease in this former premature baby. Therefore, measuring oxygen saturation during sleep would be the most appropriate next step.

168) E) The history, physical exam, and x-ray findings make pneumonia secondary to tuberculosis the most likely diagnosis compared to the other choices. Typical tuberculosis characteristics include fever, weight loss, fatigue, prolonged coughing, and lymphadenopathy. Lab findings would include monocytosis. Chest x-ray should exhibit perihilar infiltrates and hilar adenopathy.

169) C) Placement of a PPD would be the least invasive and most efficient method to confirm a diagnosis of tuberculosis. In children over age 5, IGRAs (T-spot and Quantiferon assays) are more invasive but also more specific options.

170) B) Once again, a good rule of thumb is that whenever something is in quotes the diagnosis should be taken with a grain of salt. In this case, the infant is probably not having "choking episodes" and the pediatrician who "did nothing" probably spent his lunch hour reassuring the mother and answering her and grandma's 279 questions.

This is most likely nasal congestion, commonly seen in infants, and nothing more than reassurance is necessary. Therefore no need to wake him up and you can let the doctor continue his "sleep study".

171) D) Whenever the word "pneumonia" is in quotes this is a hint that it is being defined by the parent and is not the actual diagnosis, which is probably benign, post-tussive, and emissive. Recurrent "pneumonia" with wheezing is most likely reactive airway disease. Recurrent otitis media in and of itself would not suggest an immunological disorder. However, more than one hospitalization in a child this young for "febrile pneumonia" would suggest an immunological disorder. Because of the hospitalizations you could assume that this was a pneumonia confirmed with lab, clinical, and radiological findings.

172) A) Definitive diagnosis of choanal atresia is by CT scan. The inability to pass an NG tube is only suggestive of the diagnosis.

Choanal atresia is a component of CHARGE association, which stands for coloboma, heart disease, choanal atresia, retardation, and genital and ear anomalies.

Infants are obligate nose breathers until the age of 5 months, and obstruction of both nares can be life threatening. Therefore, an oropharyngeal airway can help facilitate mouth breathing.

ANSWERS: Pulmonary

173) C) A diagnosis of asthma is supported by an FEV_1 decrease of at least 15%. When reading the question make sure they are describing a 15% decrease in **FEV_1**.

174) C) Inhaled corticosteroids used prophylactically help reduced asthma flare-ups by several mechanisms including the following:

Induce production of beta 2 receptor enhancing action of beta 2 agonists such as albuterol

Decrease the number mast cells in cells lining airway

50% of patients well controlled on inhaled steroids *still* experience exercise induced asthma

With an inhaler, without a spacer, up to 80% of the inhaled dose is deposited in the oropharynx

Leukocyte protease inhibitor synthesis is **increased.**

175) A) Remember that "diagnosed by parents" in quotes often means it is a red herring. The history is consistent with recurrent reactive airway disease.

What the mother describes as "pneumonia" isn't necessarily pneumonia. Recurrent pneumonia described by the parents is often reactive airway disease.

The history is not consistent with a diagnosis of cystic fibrosis, absence of secretory component of IgA, or foreign body aspiration.

176) A) Pulmonary function testing will confirm that it is the peak expiratory flow rate or the forced expiratory volume in one second (FEV_1) that is decreased with asthma.

177) **A)** Levalbuterol has not been proven to be superior to racemic albuterol as a first line bronchodilator in routine asthma exacerbations. Viral infections are implicated much more commonly as triggers than bacterial infections.

Regarding patients having a supply of systemic steroids at home, there are situations where this would be appropriate. Patients who have a history of repeated severe exacerbations can have a supply at home. In such cases starting treatment early has benefits provided it is done in coordination with the doctor.

Chest physical therapy and mucolytics have no role in the routine management of asthma exacerbations.

178) **D)** Inflammation is the underlying abnormality present in patients who have even mild asthma.

Inhaled cromolyn prevents both the early and late airway response to *allergy triggered* asthma and inhaled steroids help inhibit the early but not the late bronchospastic response.

Severe early bronchospasm responds promptly to short acting bronchodilators.

Mast cell activation is responsible for the *immediate* bronchospastic response to allergen exposure.

179) **D)** The most likely cause of malaise, low grade fever, headache, dry cough and bilateral patchy infiltrates on x-ray would be mycoplasma pneumonia.

Cardiology

180) **D)** The 4 components of Tetralogy of Fallot include:
1) Pulmonary stenosis
2) Right ventricular hypertrophy
3) Overriding aorta
4) VSD

Tricuspid atresia is not part of the tetralogy of Fallot.

ANSWERS: Cardiology

181)
1) E - Ventricular Fibrillation. This is the classic, disorganized nonfunctional heartbeat.
2) F - Ventricular Tachycardia.
3) G - Wolf Parkinson White syndrome. There is a short PR interval making for the classic "Delta wave."[15]
4) A - Sinus arrhythmia. This is due to an inconsistent rate of impulse coming from the sinus node.
5) C - 2nd degree AV block. Here there is a prolonged PR interval followed by dropped ventricular beats.
6) D - 3rd degree AV block. Here no impulses get through to the ventricle.
7) H - Premature ventricular contraction.
8) B - Supraventricular tachycardia.

182)
1) D
2) E
3) G
4) A
5) F
6) C
7) H
8) B

The murmur heard in **pulmonary stenosis** is distinguished from aortic stenosis and Still's murmur by the presence of an **ejection click that varies with respiration**.

Aortic stenosis is associated with a **systolic ejection click that does not vary with respiration.**

With **coarctation of the aorta, a continuous murmur over the back can be heard with long-standing disease and development of collateral flow**.

The murmur of **mitral insufficiency** is **holosystolic, heard best at the apex**. The murmur can *radiate to the axillae and the back* and can mimic the murmur of a ventricular septal defect.

---

[15] Yes, the other Delta wave is what you see on a balcony during Mardi gras, usually after a few drinks.

183) C) Disorders causing cyanotic heart disease begin with a T, but do not expect a fastball down the middle. Thus, d-Transposition and anomalous (total) pulmonary venous return both start with a T. However they may not make it that obvious on the exam.

In order to take advantage of this mnemonic you must change d-Transposition to plain old transposition of the great arteries. Anomalous (total) pulmonary venous return must be changed the more familiar Total anomalous pulmonary venous return.

Aortic insufficiency is not associated with cyanotic heart disease it does not start with a T no matter how you manipulate it.

184) C) A medium-pitched, vibratory or "musical", relatively short, systolic ejection murmur that is heard best along the left lower and midsternal border is a description of the most common innocent murmur.

185) E) A **left axis deviation** can be seen with
- Coarctation of the aorta
- AV canal defects
- Tricuspid atresia,
- Double outlet right ventricle,
- Normal heart (sometimes)

With a hypertrophic cardiomyopathy, one would have an increased left ventricular mass; however, *one would not expect to see a left axis deviation on EKG.*

Tricuspid atresia and AV canal will often have left axis deviation despite no left ventricular hypertrophy due to the aberrant conducting system. AV canal may also have a "NW" or "Superior" QRS axis of 30 to -90 degrees.

ANSWERS: Cardiology

186) A) This child is *acyanotic*, so the diagnosis won't be one of the cyanotic heart diseases, which begin with a "T" (ruling out tetralogy of Fallot and transposition of the great vessels).

Children with anomalous coronary arteries present with symptoms of myocardial infarction, not cardiac murmurs.

This narrows us down to two choices ASD and VSD.

The clinical scenario including the description of a holosystolic murmur is most consistent with an infant with a large VSD that is going into heart failure.

187) D) The gold standard for diagnosing subacute bacterial endocarditis would be a blood culture. This is an example where it is important to focus on what is being asked (also called "reading the question") and not jumps to instinct in picking 24-hour EKG.

Echocardiogram, would also *not be the best answer*. Although it may identify vegetations, this in and of itself would not rule out bacterial endocarditis.

Had the question been phrased differently—asking the most diagnostic *cardiac* study—then cardiac echo would be the correct answer. Always read the question and circle the key words so they stand out.

188) C) Truncus arteriosus is characterized by a large ventricular septal defect over which a large, single great vessel (truncus) arises. This single great vessel carries blood both to the body and to the lungs.

Therefore the pulmonary artery and the aorta combine for one vessel with partially saturated blood and equal pressure. Since both ventricles are essentially contiguous you have the same pressure and saturation seen in the truncus (combined vessel)

The pulmonary vein and left atrium are largely unaffected and their pressure and saturation is the same as you would see in a normal heart.

The key to answering this correctly is the same pressures and saturations in the common truncus, RV and LV.

189) C) This cardiac catheterization demonstrates

- Increased saturations on the right side of the heart equal to the left (which is less than normal)

- Increased pressure in all chambers and gradients on the right side and decreased pressure in all chambers and gradients on the left side.

This is consistent with total anomalous pulmonary venous return where none of the four veins that drain blood from the lungs to the heart is attached to the left atrium. In TAPVR, oxygenated blood returns to the right atrium instead.

190) C) In addition to coronary aneurysms, cardiac complications also include myocarditis and valvulitis. High dose aspirin is used during the acute phase until fever subsides.

Following this, low dose aspirin is continued for several weeks or until the platelet count returns to normal.

Coronary aneurysms start developing early in the disease but they do not manifest immediately. Therefore cardiac echo done at the time of diagnosis is to assess for myocarditis which may not have manifested clinically yet.

IV gamma globulin is given during the **acute** phase.

191) C) The history and presentation of this patient is consistent with costochondritis. Their noting that the grandfather died of an MI at 65 and the father is being treated for hypertension are decoys. Cardiac disease in relatives older than 55 would not reflect a risk for cardiac disease in a young person. There is no evidence for GERD causing the chest pain.

There is no history of abdominal pain and the physical exam is benign. The unremarkable physical exam does not rule out costochondritis either. It might have resolved by the time the patient got to the doctor's office.

192) C) The most appropriate first step would be to measure serum triglycerides and cholesterol before moving on to any therapeutic modalities.

Cardiac echo and stress test would be premature at this point.

Heme Onc

193) C) Clotting factor 8 is not vitamin K dependent. Memorize the vitamin K dependent factors, 2, 7, 9 and 10; they always ask this. There is nothing more to it than that.

194) C) Pre-B cell type is the most common subtype and the one with the best prognosis. Rapid initial response to treatment also corresponds to a good prognosis.

195) A) With a child with **unilateral disease** the chances are roughly **5%** that another child will have the disease; with **bilateral disease** the chances jump to **50%.**

196) E) An exchange transfusion *can* reduce the incidence of stroke, which occurs in 6% of patients with sickle cell disease. CVAs are due to both small and large vessel injury and focal strokes can result in subtle neuropsychological deficits. However, MRI, not CT, provides the most accurate diagnostic assessment by providing better image resolution. MRI also is more sensitive in identifying subtle parenchymal changes common just after a stroke has occurred.

197) D) Neutrophils are the first line of defense of skin and mucous membranes against the rest of the world while fungal and other infections may occur. The best answer is choice D skin and GI flora. Treatment in the face of fever and other toxic signs in a neutropenic patient should be directed toward these organisms.

Likewise if they were to ask what the most common way neutropenia presents is, the correct answer is oral mucosal ulcerations and gingivitis.

198) D) If you are given no other information then viral syndrome is the most likely cause of neutropenia for a patient in your practice.

199) 1) (C)
2) (B)
3) (A)
4) (D)

In **iron deficiency anemia,** the **TIBC** is high. Think of iron binding capacity as "trucks" to transport iron where it is needed. When there isn't a lot of iron around, as is the case with iron deficiency anemia, there are plenty of truck waiting around and the iron binding capacity is high. Serum iron stores or serum ferritin is low in iron deficiency anemia.

However, with **anemia of chronic illness,** there isn't a lot of iron around. The trucks don't have any gas and they remain in the garage, so the iron binding capacity is low. Since the reserves were there before the illness, **serum ferritin** is high in anemia of chronic illness.

It is easy to distinguish thalassemia from iron deficiency anemia. The RDW will be high in iron deficiency and low in thalassemia

Serum **FEP** (free erythrocyte protoporphyrin) is elevated in both **lead poisoning** and **iron deficiency.** However, TIBC is elevated in iron deficiency and decreased in lead poisoning.

200) 1) (A)
2) (B)
3) (A)
4) (D)
5) (B)
6) (D)

G6PD deficiency is an X-linked recessive disorder that is associated with **Heinz bodies.**

Howell-Jolly bodies are associated with sickle cell disease.

While hereditary spherocytosis is an example of a hemolytic anemia, it can also be associated with an **aplastic crisis** in association with a **parvoviral infection.**

ANSWERS: Heme One

201)
1) (C)
2) (D)
3) (D)
4) (A)
5) (B)
6) (D)

Thrombocytopenia is seen in both Wiskott Aldrich Syndrome (WAS) and Idiopathic thrombocytopenic purpura (ITP).

Eczema is only seen in Wiskott Aldrich syndrome.

Only ITP can be seen following a recent viral illness.

Increased PTT, abnormal platelet *function* and increased risk for malignancies are not seen in ITP or WAS.

202)
1) (A)
2) (B)
3) (A)
4) (B)
5) (D)

Joint pain is typically associated with JRA.

However, **bone pain**, lymphadenopathy and hepatosplenomegaly are more typical of leukemia. The increased incidence of leukemia with exposure to microwave towers has never been proven, so this is another popularly held myth that might steer you wrong on the Boards.

203) D) Whenever you are presented with a child who was "delivered at home," you have to assume that Vitamin K IM was not given. In addition the infant is 12 days old and has not been examined by a physician yet. You must consider hemorrhagic disease of the newborn up there on the differential, or sepsis if they present you with a scenario consistent with it.

In this case, the most likely diagnosis is *hemorrhagic disease of the newborn.*

A moderate decrease of the vitamin K-dependent factors[16] normally occurs in all newborn infants by 48 to 72 hours after birth. This transient deficiency of vitamin K-dependent factors probably is due largely to the absence of bacterial intestinal flora normally responsible for synthesis of vitamin K. In addition, **breast milk is a poor source of vitamin K,** and hemorrhagic complications have appeared more commonly in breast-fed than in formula-fed infants.

This is one of the few cases where formula would have an "advantage" over breast milk. This classic form of hemorrhagic disease of the newborn is responsive to vitamin K therapy.

Henoch Schönlein purpura is unlikely in this age group and with this presentation.

The blue areas of discoloration that are supposed to make you suspect child abuse are, of course, nothing more than Mongolian spots.

204) C) **While Fanconi's anemia is a congenital disorder, the pancytopenia typically isn't noted until the child is older than 3.** It is inherited in an autosomal recessive pattern. In addition to affecting blood cells, the disease affects the skeletal system[17] and results in abnormal skin pigmentation and kidney abnormalities.

Fanconi's anemia is also associated with chromosomal fragility leading to an increased risk of transformation to AML or myelodysplastic syndrome and with short stature.

205) D) The classic presentation of neuroblastoma in childhood would be an abdominal mass, perhaps coupled with raccoon eyes (periorbital ecchymoses). However, the tumor can also appear in the mediastinum. Neuroblastomas are tumors of the sympathetic chain. When it appears in this area of the body, the tumor can cause compression of the recurrent laryngeal nerve and the cervical sympathetic chain, resulting in Horner's syndrome.

---

[16] Factors II, VII, IX, and X. memorize these; it is frequently tested on the exam.
[17] Hypoplastic thumbs and aplasia of the radius.

ANSWERS: Heme One

206) B) *Iron deficiency anemia* is a microcytic anemia; therefore, the MCV will be reduced. **Both the serum ferritin levels and the serum iron levels are reduced.**[18]

In iron deficiency anemia, the serum iron binding capacity is actually increased, not reduced. The treatment of course is with iron supplementation.

207) B) Given that 22 light years is a distance and not a period of time, this is easily ruled out. Cyclic neutropenia is characterized by regularly recurring episodes of neutropenia, typically lasting 3-6 days. In between these neutropenic episodes is a period of about 3 weeks.

This is similar to the timing and duration of menstrual cycles, which should help you remember this otherwise difficult fact.

These patients can present with oral ulcers and lesions, as well as adenopathy. They may also present with chronic periodontitis.

Consider this diagnosis carefully when presented with a patient presenting with unusual pathogens such as *Clostridium perfringens*.

208) E) Burr[19] and Helmet cells, as well as schistocytes, are all associated with hemolysis, as seen in hemolytic uremic syndrome.

Aaron Burr was the 3rd vice president of the U.S. who is better known for challenging Alexander Hamilton to a duel and mortally wounding him. Alexander Hamilton however has been immortalized on the $10 bill.

You can remember that schistocytes are associated with hemolytic uremic syndrome by picturing Aaron burr "shisting" a sword into Alexander Hamilton's kidney. Picture Burr wearing a "helmet" to remember that helmet cells are also associated with hemolytic uremic syndrome.

Of course, thrombocytopenia is an integral part of hemolytic uremic syndrome.

The **Coombs test** *can be* positive when hemolytic uremic syndrome is caused by pneumococcus, but **it is not positive with "typical" hemolytic uremic syndrome.** Again, reading the question for key words is important.

---

[18] Note that in the anemia of chronic illness the serum iron level is reduced but the serum ferritin level is increased.
[19] Okay so it isn't really Aaron Burr cells. We took poetic license for the sake of humor.

209) C) This is a normocytic anemia making iron deficiency anemia unlikely. Folate deficiency is a macrocytic anemia and therefore also unlikely.

The high reticulocyte count findings and the fact that this child is African American places sickle cell anemia high on the differential.

Therefore hemoglobin electrophoresis would certainly be the most logical next step in establishing the correct diagnosis.

210) E) Severe anemia, hypersplenism, growth retardation, and chronic fatigue could all be indications for a transfusion. Extramedullary hematopoiesis however could be an indication for a splenectomy.

211) E) Elevated serum unconjugated bilirubin elevated lactic dehydrogenase, and low serum haptoglobin levels would be seen in any hemolytic anemia. Spherocytes can be seen in any case of immune mediated hemolysis including ABO incompatibility. In the case of ABO incompatibility, the direct Coombs would be positive, but it is negative in hereditary spherocytosis.

212) E) Females and younger age at diagnosis are both factors which increase the risk of cardiotoxicity in children on anthracycline. Cardiotoxicity can occur with relatively lower doses.

However screening is done every 1-5 years depending on *cumulative dose.*

213) B) Secondary malignancies are especially common in survivors of Hodgkin's lymphoma. They are at particular risk for developing AML, Non Hodgkin's lymphoma and breast cancer.

ANSWERS: Renal

214) E) The history and presentation is consistent with a diagnosis of G6PD deficiency with the antibiotic (usually a sulfa or nitrofurantoin) serving as the oxidative stress.

215) A) Wilms tumor typically presents as a painless abdominal mass often in an asymptomatic patient. Typically it is noted by the parent while dressing or bathing the child

216) B) A child with painless abdominal pain along with systemic symptoms especially the periorbital ecchymoses "raccoon eyes" leads us to neuroblastoma as the most likely diagnosis.

217) E) There are no absolute hemoglobin or hematocrit levels that trigger consideration for a blood transfusion. Clinical conditions drive the decision. However Estimated traumatic blood loss or surgical blood loss of 15% would be considered triggers for a blood transfusion in the absence of physiological compensation.

Renal

218) D) **P**ost –strep glomerulonephritis, **m**embranoproliferative glomerulonephritis, and **s**ystemic lupus nephritis all are associated with low serum complement levels. Because if you have "P-M-S" you would not be in the mood to "compliment" anyone.

219) D) There is nothing in the history to suggest any specific cause other than essential hypertension in this patient. Essential hypertension often runs in families, which is the reason the father's and the uncle's histories are mentioned.

By the way if they had not noted that the blood pressure was elevated on 3 separate occasions, preferably one month apart, it is not hypertension by definition.

220) B) Prune belly syndrome more commonly affects males, and cryptorchidism is one of the associated findings that can be seen. While the urethral and vaginal structures can be involved in females, **ovarian dysplasia is not seen in prune belly syndrome**. Renal dysplasia and pulmonary hypoplasia are also typically seen.

221) D) This question is another example where writing down the meaning of the lab values in words is critical. In addition, when presented with the components of the anion gap, you need to calculate and note whether it is elevated.

Here the Bicarb is low and you are therefore dealing with a **metabolic acidosis**. If there were a respiratory component, you would have been provided with blood gas values. The sodium, potassium, and chloride are normal. The anion gap would be (136-114-10) = 12. The anion gap is within the normal range.

A normal anion gap rules out organic acids as the cause of the metabolic acidosis. There is no indication of genetic short stature since they do not mention the parents' heights, and they wouldn't give all these lab values if that were the diagnosis. Polycystic renal disease does not result in metabolic acidosis at all, so this choice is eliminated.

You are now down to proximal and distal renal tubular acidosis. Often, but not always, if you have these two diagnoses among the choices, it will likely come down to one of them. This is a general rule; however, there are occasionally exceptions to this rule.

The key to distinguishing these two is the pH of the urine. Distal tubular acidosis is the inability to dump hydrogen ions into the urine. Therefore, a pH >5.5, in light of the severity of the acidosis, makes distal tubular acidosis the most likely diagnosis.[20]

222) B) The clinical scenario described is that of nephrotic syndrome, and since **minimal change nephrotic syndrome is the most common cause of nephrotic syndrome, this is the most likely diagnosis**. Focal segmental glomerulonephritis is the second most common cause of nephrotic syndrome. Lupus nephritis is a disease more common in adolescents, not in a child of 4. Therefore, it is important to pay attention to the age of the child presented when considering the differential diagnosis.

There is nothing in the vignette to indicate liver failure or a diagnosis of Henoch-Schönlein purpura.

---

[20] Distal renal tubular acidosis results in nephrocalcinosis. If they note increased echogenicity on renal ultrasound, this would be another indication that distal renal tubular acidosis is the diagnosis.

ANSWERS: Renal

223) B) Given the alkaline pH of the urine, the most likely etiology is proteus since proteus contains an enzyme that produces ammonia from urea. An additional finding they could describe would be a "foul odor".

224) D) All of the choices can be associated with and/or result in hemolytic uremic syndrome **with the exception of an X-linked recessive inheritance pattern**. Indeed, both oral contraceptives and pregnancy can result in hemolytic uremic syndrome.

There is an inheritance pattern associated with hemolytic uremic syndrome, but it is an **autosomal recessive or dominant**, not an X-linked inheritance pattern. You should consider this choice if they present you with a classic case of hemolytic uremic syndrome presenting in siblings over a period of time. If you really want to get technical,[21] it is believed that the inherited form of hemolytic uremic syndrome is due to *Factor H deficiency* of the "alternative pathway" of complement.[22]

225) C) The most ominous sign of glomerular disease is casts containing RBCs, not serrated or dysmorphic RBCs. The presence of dysmorphic RBCs does, however, *suggest* glomerular disease, but *the absence does not rule it out*. Regarding choice E, a "spot" urine calcium/creatinine check is sufficient to rule out hypercalciuria as a cause of hematuria; a 24-hour sample is not needed.

226) D) Calcium, Oxalate, struvite and cystine can be seen on plain film x-ray, uric acid stones cannot.

Cystine stones are only faintly radiopaque but this is the boards.

227) C) Helical nonenhanced CT is superior to IVP and other studies in offering the highest sensitivity and specificity in identifying small stones. Other diagnoses in the differential likewise can be identified with this study.

---

[21] Or want to score high and not just pass like the rest of us.
[22] Whatever that is; I can hardly remember the "traditional" pathway of complement, let alone the alternative. I would look it up except the cloud of dust enveloping the book might trigger a hyperacute case of hemolytic uremic syndrome right on the spot, and it isn't worth the risk.

228) C) Recurrent nephrolithiasis is the only clinical manifestation of cystinuria, However in addition to cystine stones it can, albeit rarely, be associated with calcium oxalate stones.

Treatment includes increased fluid intake and alkalinization of urine.

Cystinuria is distinct from cystinosis which is a lysosomal storage disease which is not associated with renal stones.

229) E) Oligohydramnios and bilateral hydronephrosis would be consistent with prune belly syndrome and posterior urethral valves. Note that posterior urethral valves are more common and would be correct if you had to make one choice only.

230) D) Hypertension in a teenager needs to be addressed. Since the elevated blood pressure was documented on 3 separate occasions by 3 different nurses, by definition hypertension exists. The best initial treatment is weight loss often with a nutrition consult and exercise.

Urinary

231) D) Ocular chlamydia infection and chlamydia pneumonia in the newborn period can be obtained during the birth process.

However, a chlamydia vaginal infection in a pre-adolescent girl is almost always due to sexual abuse.

Malodorous vaginal discharge is frequently due to a foreign body (for example, toilet paper);

Anterior hymenal tears may not necessarily be due to sexual abuse. Tissue missing above the 3-9 O'clock position or the anterior position is a common normal variant. Therefore what may be described as a hymenal tear may actually be missing tissue within the context of this being a normal variant. Posterior hymenal tear is more likely to be due to sexual abuse.

Molluscum contagiosum is a benign skin lesion in children; bacterial vaginosis can be seen following sexual abuse but it is nonspecific because it can be the result of rubbing in the genital area.

ANSWERS: Urinary

232) D) The symptoms are consistent with **torsion of the appendix testes.** It typically presents in a child between 2-11 years of age. The inflammation typically resolves within 3-10 days, and **surgical intervention is typically not indicated.**

233) D) If one simply followed the "least invasive procedure is usually correct" rule, it would have been simple enough to select the correct answer. Since the physical examination is normal an MRI study is unnecessary.

Since there is no mention of nocturnal enuresis, DDAVP therapy on a PRN basis is not necessary. DDAVP is reserved for occasional use when staying dry overnight is absolutely necessary for social reasons, for example a sleep over at a friend's house.

Since this child was toilet trained and assumed to be fully continent for the past year, the most likely diagnosis and first thing to be ruled out would be a urinary tract infection; therefore, a urinalysis would be the most appropriate next step.

234) D) The only explanation for bilateral, painless scrotal swelling which transilluminates, in an infant would be hydrocele.

235) E) A foreign body is commonly responsible for vaginal bleeding in preadolescent females particularly if it is described as malodorous.

In this patient, the foul-smelling discharge makes a vaginal foreign body, such as toilet paper, the most likely explanation.

236) C) In up to 1/3 of cases Henoch Schönlein purpura can present with acute pain, erythema and swelling of the scrotum especially in boys younger than 7.

Henpecked shoreline purpura is beyond the scope of this discussion indeed.

Neurology

237) A) Lisch nodules, neurofibromas, learning disabilities, and optic gliomas are associated with NF type 1. Additional findings include boney defects such as intramedullary fibrosis, cortical thinning and sphenoid bone dysplasia.

However acoustic neuromas are associated with neurofibromatosis **type 2.**

238) C) While it is safe to reassure parents that a child experiencing a simple febrile seizure stands little chance of developing epilepsy, the chances of developing epilepsy are slightly higher for a child who has suffered a complex febrile seizure and this is felt to be due to a genetic predisposition.

Therefore while the risk is still low it does double from 1 to 2%. Fair? Not really but who said board exams are fair?

The risk of epilepsy is irrespective of the number of febrile seizures the child experiences. Therefore choice C is NOT true. Neuroimaging is rarely indicated and lytes, glucose and even calcium should be reserved for cases accompanied by diarrhea.

While an "LP" isn't routinely indicated, meningitis must be ruled out "clinically" and if there is clinical evidence of meningitis an LP *would be appropriate.*

239) E) This is a typical description of partial complex seizures. School aged children are typically affected, and the episodes can start out with "staring spells", which then generalize and lead to "automatisms" such as clicking sounds. Family history can be negative, and EEGs are frequently negative. Treatment is with anticonvulsants.

Rolandic seizures typically occur at night, which helps differentiate them from partial complex seizures.

Absence seizures do not occur with automatisms and do not typically result in a post ictal picture. In addition, there are typical EEG findings. Therefore, if there is a negative EEG in the question, you can usually cross out absence seizures from the choices presented.

ANSWERS: Neurology

240) D) There is no evidence of trauma so subdural and epidural hematomas are ruled out.

Cardiomegaly and failure to thrive suggest congestive heart failure.

This would make a **vein of Galen malformation**.

Consider this diagnosis when they describe an infant with hydrocephalus and congestive heart failure.

241)
1) (B)
2) (C)
3) (A)
4) (D)

Absence seizures are associated with a 3 per second spike and wave EEG pattern.

Infantile spasms are associated with a hypsarrhythmia pattern on EEG.

Complex partial seizures would be associated with a child presenting with lip smacking.

Rolandic seizures typically occur at night and this should be part of the clinical description on the boards.

This can be remembered by picturing a child with rolandic seizures **rolling out of bed at night.**

242)
1) (A)
2) (F)
3) (B)
4) (D)
5) (E)
6) (C)

Chorea can be described as smooth movements of the extremities.

Rapid rhythmic movements would be a tremor.

Twisting, assuming postures would be a **dystonia.**

Brief muscle jerking movements would be **myoclonus**.

Brief movements of the face and shoulder would be a **tic.**

Excessive ants-in-the-pants-like movements would be a classic description of **hyperactivity.**

243) E) The clinical presentation is most consistent with a cerebral hemorrhage due to an *arteriovenous malformations* resulting from a failure of normal capillary bed development between arteries and veins during embryogenesis. Arteriovenous malformations produce abnormal shunting of blood, causing an expansion of vessels and a space-occupying effect or rupture of a vein and intracerebral bleeding. Arteriovenous malformations are typically located in the cerebral hemisphere.

Rupture of arteriovenous malformations causes a severe headache, vomiting, and nuchal rigidity due to subarachnoid bleeding, progressive hemiparesis, and a focal or generalized seizure.

244) A) Myasthenia gravis typically presents with bulbar[23] and systemic weakness.

Multiple sclerosis would not typically present in this age group and neither would "infantile" botulism. **Polio** is rare and they would have to give you a clue such as lack of immunization and/or recent travel to a place where polio is endemic. Guillain-Barré presents with ascending[24] paralysis typically following a viral illness.

245) B) The presence of anti-acetylcholine antibodies causes the disease. A positive edrophonium chloride (Tensilon®) test and EMG findings are diagnostic.

246) E) A cholinesterase-inhibiting drug (anticholinesterases) such as neostigmine or pyridostigmine is critical in managing the symptoms of this disorder.

247) B) This is a typical description of *infantile spasms,* known previously by the politically incorrect term "salaam movements". This "visual", however, remains a simple way to recognize the presentation of infantile spasms. Keep in mind that infantile spasms may also present with tuberous sclerosis, so watch out for a description of both in the same patient.

The hypsarrhythmic pattern on EEG[25] is also characteristic of infantile spasms and gives away the diagnosis. Treatment is with ACTH.

---

[23] By bulbar we are not referring to light bulbs. We are referring to bulbar weakness of the muscles innervated by the cranial nerves, manifesting in decreased extraocular eye movements, diminished gag reflex, and laryngeal muscle weakness.

[24] Legs first, and then "ascending" up to the face.

[25] Not to worry, you won't be presented with the actual pattern; you will just need to recognize the word.

ANSWERS: Neurology

248) C) With depressed consciousness and continued deviation of both eyes, this would likely be due to persistent seizure activity and should be treated as such.

249) E) The combination of a transient focal headache with contralateral weakness would be consistent with a diagnosis of familial hemiplegic migraine. This is supported by the family history of migraine headaches.

250) B) A tic disorder would be characterized by a motor **or** vocal tic but not both. Sniffing which cannot be suppressed would be considered to be a *vocal tic* as would chirping sounds or throat clearing.

Children with Tourette syndrome have *both* motor and vocal tics, not necessarily at the same time but they both must be present to establish the diagnosis. They must occur daily for one year with no tic free period longer than 3 months.

Since the boy is alert during these episodes this cannot be absence seizures. There is nothing to suggest attention deficit hyperactivity disorder.

Although the boy is sniffing there is nothing to suggest allergic rhinitis. The eye blinking would constitute a motor tic. Therefore the combination of a motor and vocal tic would suggest a diagnosis of Tourette syndrome.

251) C) Children with epilepsy may take a bath or swim provided there is an adult supervision. Driving is permitted provided the patient has been seizure free for 3-12 months.

Obtaining an EEG is not useful in weaning a patient off of medications. The presence or absence of seizure activity is more important.

Juvenile myoclonic epilepsy requires lifetime treatment.

252) D) Onset of seizure before age 1 and a low degree of fever at the onset of the seizure increase the chances of having febrile seizures in the future. However they do not increase the risk for developing epilepsy.

However a family history of epilepsy places a child at increased risk of developing epilepsy. In this case, a "febrile seizure" may just be the first seizure, triggered by a febrile illness. In addition a child experiencing a complex febrile seizure would be at increased risk for developing epilepsy. The following factors would constitute a complex febrile seizure:

· Duration longer than 15 minutes
· Recurrence within 24 hours
· Focal seizure

Musculoskeletal

253) D) While this is an X-linked disorder, it is not always inherited from the mother. Since X-linked recessive disorder is one of the other choices it may seem like the two are contradictory. Following the rule to never choose a question with "always" in it, you will likely get this correct.

This is a disease with a high spontaneous mutation rate. **In up to 1/3 of the cases the mother is *not* the carrier.**

254) C) Since this is a girl where less than 2 years of growth is expected and the angle is less than 25 degrees, only watchful observation is needed and a follow-up film in 6 months.

255) C) This is a classic description of dermatomyositis and the treatment is with steroids.

ANSWERS: Musculoskeletal

256) A) A Salter-Harris I injury is a disruption of the growth plate only. It is a diagnosis often made on clinical grounds since the fracture can be quite subtle. Therefore, it is very likely that the injury from several months earlier was a Salter-Harris I fracture that was not diagnosed and this is a re-injury.

Conversion disorder? I don't think so!

257) D) Each of the signs listed are common findings with TMJ dysfunction except for swelling of the TMJ. Consider that snapping your gum excessively can also lead to TMJ dysfunction.

Excessive discussion of board questions with colleagues after you have already taken the exam can also lead to TMJ dysfunction followed by conversion reaction.

258) B) SCFE is the slippage of the epiphysis of the proximal femur in relation to the metaphysis. For those who do not feel comfortable with orthopedic Latin, this is simply the slippage of the femoral head. It often appears as an ice cream scoop slipping off the cone on x-ray, especially on the Boards.

SCFE often presents as referred knee pain, especially on the exam. Estrogen increases the strength of the growth plate, and both testosterone and growth hormone weaken the plate.

Therefore, elevated estrogen levels would not be a contributing factor. SCFE occurs more frequently in males and in African-Americans. Obesity is another significant risk factor.

259) E) **Osteogenic sarcoma** and **Ewing's sarcoma** are not benign tumors.

Osteoid osteoma, while common on the Boards, is not the most common benign tumor seen in children.

Osteochondromas are outgrowths of normal bone as well as cartilage and are the most common benign tumors in children. These are confirmed on x-ray and removed when symptomatic or when risk for malignant transformation is present. Malignant transformation should be suspected when continued growth occurs after skeletal maturity is reached or there is a new onset of pain.

Osgood Schlatter's disease is caused by micro-fractures of the tibial tuberosity and is not a bone tumor.

260) B) Children with **achondroplasia** have normal intelligence. It can be inherited in an autosomal dominant fashion, although most cases arise from a new mutation to normal parents. Therefore, genetic testing is not always performed or necessary. While virtually all infants and children with this disorder are born with relatively large heads, only a fraction have true hydrocephalus.

Lumbar spinal stenosis can present later in life, and loss of bladder and bowel control may be a an eventual complication.

261) E) Bilateral lower leg pain occurring exclusively at night in the absence of daytime symptoms, systemic symptoms or physical findings is classic for growing pains and requires nothing more than reassurance.

262) C) Legg calve Perthes disease is a self limited disease resulting from avascular necrosis of the capital femoral epiphysis. It frequently occurs in boys between ages 4-10. Onset before the age of 6 carries a better prognosis due to the extended period of time for bone remodeling.

Girls tend to have a higher prevalence of bilateral disease. However bilateral disease is not associated with more severe disease or a worse prognosis.

MRI is more helpful than x-ray during the early stages of disease.

263) C) The classic history of slipped capital femoral epiphysis (SCFE) is a teenager, usually obese who presents with a history of minor trauma, with symptoms out of proportion to the trauma.

Although SCFE involves the hip joint, pain is often refereed to the knee. They present with the leg externally rotated and slightly flexed. Passive internal rotation is difficult due to pain

264) E) Idiopathic scoliosis is due to multiple factors and does not follow any specific inheritance patterns.

ANSWERS: Musculoskeletal

265) D) The appropriate order of diagnostic testing for Duchenne muscular dystrophy is

Creatinine kinase levels → genetic analysis → muscle biopsy

Clearly muscle biopsy is the most invasive and is last. Creatinine kinase levels would be a first initial screen. Molecular genetic analysis has advanced in recent years. These have reduced the number of patients receiving muscle biopsy unnecessarily.

A muscle biopsy would not be useful if creatinine kinase levels and genetic analysis are normal.

266) A) Are you getting the picture? More often than not, the correct answer will be multifactorial when this is among the choices. This is not a hard rule and of course; if you know that another choice is the answer then pick that one.

However, when in doubt, pick multifactorial as the answer.

267) D) The conservative or non surgical intervention of choice to treat congenital talipes equinovarus is casting and splinting.

Dermatology

268)
1) (D) - Tinea capitis
2) (E) - Alopecia areata
3) (C) - Trichotillomania
4) (B) - Alopecia totalis
5) (A) - Alopecia neurotica.

On the exam tinea capitis will often be described as scalp inflammation and **black dots.**

Alopecia areata will be described as complete areas of smooth hair loss with no inflammation or discoloration.

Trichotillomania is incomplete patches of hair loss with hair shafts of varying lengths caused by hair pulling.

Alopecia totalis as the name implies, means "total baldness" in Latin. Therefore even the eyebrows and eyelashes are involved.

Alopecia neurotica is baldness as a result of being totally neurotic and hyper such as a pediatrician going from a total head of hair to total baldness while preparing for the boards. This is also known as "Board Pattern Baldness".

269) E) This is a classic description of tinea pedis, or "athlete's foot". The fact that the sibling has it is a red herring set to throw you off the trail toward thinking the diagnosis is scabies. However there is nothing else in the history to suggest this.

Hyperhidrosis[26] would explain the foul odor but not the other physical findings described. Tinea pedis in and of itself does not result in a foul odor. However, a moist environment in the shoes would lead to a foul odor akin to a damp basement in the summertime.

270) E) Erythema infectiosum, which is the rash associated with fifth disease, can be described as a "slapped cheek" appearance along with a reticular rash on the extremities. Human parvovirus B19 is felt to be the etiological agent.

---

[26] Excessive sweating of the palms and soles in response to emotional stimuli.

ANSWERS: Dermatology

271) E) *Neisseria meningitidis* bacteremia may result in the release of an endotoxin, which can lead to DIC and deplete clotting factors and protein C. This is especially problematic in kids already deficient in Protein C.

Deficiency of protein C can lead to cutaneous infarctions called *purpura fulminans*, which is an ominous sign.

272) E) The rash described is "erythema nodosum". It is a hypersensitivity reaction that can be associated with any of the conditions listed. However, they asked for the **most likely** cause, and that would be Group A *Strep*.

273) E) In cases initially thought to be *severe seborrheic dermatitis* that do not resolve and progress to ulcerated lesions coupled with petechiae and purpura, histiocytosis X must be ruled out. This is best accomplished by skin biopsy.

274) E) The rash is a typical description of Gianotti-Crosti syndrome. It is often associated with viral infections, including EBV, hepatitis B, and CMV, among others.

If you picked erythema erythema you would be red red in the face with embarrassment.

275) A) Baseline laboratory studies are not necessary when griseofulvin is given to children. Topical antifungal agents are not effective because the fungus of tinea capitis resides within the hair shafts, *not on them*. However, topical steroids can sometimes help alleviate the inflammatory reaction seen with tinea capitis. For better absorption, it is recommended that griseofulvin be taken with lipid-containing foods.

276) C) With no papules or pustules, the treatment is aimed toward taking care of the comedones.[27] Since retinoic acid[28] is the single most effective agent in the treatment of comedonal acne, it is the correct answer. The results of retinoic acid are not seen for 3-6 months and sunscreen must be used with retinoic acid because of the increased sensitivity to sunlight. Turn out the light while waiting.

Rheumatology

277) C) Penicillin G or VK, sulfisoxazole, sulfadiazine, sulfonamides in general as well as erythromycin can all be used for preventing rheumatic fever recurrence. Cefaclor would not be effective treatment for recurrent rheumatic fever.

278) C) Recognizing that the cardiac manifestations are the most serious ones, you have probably narrowed your choices down to B and C. If you have not focused on details you will have a 50% chance of answering this incorrectly.

Remember, mitral valve insufficiency will often be the initial or only manifestation during an initial attack. However only 30% of children will have any evidence of it a year later.

On the other hand, when **aortic insufficiency** occurs, it leads to permanent damage in 90% of cases.

Therefore the most important long term concern will be aortic insufficiency rather than mitral valve insufficiency.

Rheumatic fever *never* causes *permanent* joint damage. If they state that there is a rapid relief of symptoms with salicylate administration, this is typical and a dead give away in the wording of the question. If they describe joint pain continuing past the acute phase, then the questioner is leading you to a different diagnosis.

Sydenham's chorea can last up to 15 weeks at most. The typical erythema marginatum rash is short lived.

---

[27] Dilated epithelial lined follicular sac filled with keratinous material, lipid, and bacteria; much easier to just say comedones.
[28] Tretinoin = Retin-A®

ANSWERS: Rheumatology

279) C) High persistent fever is the earliest sign, which makes it a difficult disorder to diagnose before the other signs manifest. The fever remits with treatment with IVIG and high dose aspirin.

280) D) Erythema infectiosum is another name for "Fifth Disease" which is another name for "Slapped Cheek Disease" caused by Parvovirus B19. Slap yourself on the cheek if you answer this easy question incorrectly.

Erythema marginatum is the rash that is one of the major Jones criteria.

281) 1) (C)
2) (F)
3) (D)
4) (B)
5) (E)
6) (A)

A WBC count less than 200 would be consistent with normal synovial fluid. Trauma would result in joint effusion with synovial fluid with more WBC than normal and increased viscosity and clear.

Decreased viscosity with roughly 5,000 WBC and cloudy would be consistent with a diagnosis of rheumatic fever.

JRA would present with a synovial fluid, which is cloudy with decreased viscosity with a markedly elevated WBC in the 20,000 range.

Septic arthritis would present with synovial fluid which is yellow, decreased viscosity and very high WBC in the 200,000 range.

Kendall Jackson chardonnay is fluid like septic arthritis is yellow, with bouquet with a kick and a slight after-taste, 10,000 + epithelial cells and maybe a handful of WBC's.

282)
1) (E)
2) (A)
3) (B)
4) (C)
5) (D)

Mixed connective tissue disease is associated with high titers of antibodies to an RNase-sensitive component of extractable nuclear antigen. It has some clinical features in common with JRA, SLE, and scleroderma.

In *antiphospholipid syndrome*, there are antibodies to phospholipids that cross-react with the spirochete antigen. This is the explanation for the false-positive VDRL.

Wegener's granulomatosis is due to a systemic vasculitis.

Schönlein-Henoch purpura is a result of vasculitis that is IgA mediated. When the kidneys are involved, the histopathology is identical to Berger's disease (IgA nephropathy).

Although anti-SM is only found in 30% of patients with *SLE*, when it is positive it is a reliable confirmation of a diagnosis of SLE.

283) C) While all of the choices are consistent with a variety of conditions that include hypermobility syndrome, including choice E, which is a description of William's syndrome, the vast majority of children with hypermobility syndrome have no other conditions and will not be noted by their pediatrician.

284) D) Patients with **systemic lupus erythematosus** typically have anemia of chronic illness. However, they can also have an autoimmune hemolytic anemia. Immune mediated thrombocytopenia also occurs. Leukopenia is not uncommon.

However leukocytosis is not typically seen in lupus.

ANSWERS: Ophthalmology

285) B) Neonatal lupus erythematosus is due to transplacental transfer of antibodies which can result in cutaneous lupus lesions which resolve without scarring. Hepatitis is another possible manifestation which resolves as the maternal antibodies disappear.

However congenital heart block is irreversible because it is due to permanent damage to the conducting system making placement of a permanent pacemaker necessary.

286) C) Non steroidal anti inflammatory medications are used to treat arthritis and fever in patients with lupus. Glucocorticosteroid are used in particular to treat renal, hematological, and CNS manifestations.

Sunscreen is important to protect against cutaneous manifestations. Cyclophosphamide is used particularly for renal and CNS manifestations.

Insulin is not used in treating lupus.

Ophthalmology

287) D) The most likely cause of conjunctivitis–otitis media syndrome is *H. influenzae*. You could have been diverted by their noting the immunizations being up to date. However the organism *H. influenzae* is non typeable. The Hib vaccine is against Type b.

288) B) The description of excessive tearing or watery discharge with runny nose, vague sore throat and shoddy cervical adenopathy is consistent with **viral conjunctivitis. Supportive measures would be most appropriate.**

Since there is no history of eye trauma, fluorescein staining to assess for corneal abrasion is not indicated. There is no indication for moxifloxacin eye drops and certainly not for systemic antibiotics. There should be no need for referral to an ophthalmologist.

The most common cause of viral conjunctivitis is adenovirus.

289) D) The presentation described in the question is typical of eye infection due to **Neisseria meningitidis** or **Neisseria gonorrhoeae**. It is described as acute onset of excessively purulent discharge, pseudomembrane formation and typically adenopathy most likely preauricular lymphadenopathy. Therefore, although gonorrhea could be one of the etiologies, syphilis is not, and is there merely as a diversion since it is the wrong STD. It is important to keep your STDs straight.

This would be considered to be an ophthalmological emergency and calling in the specialist would be correct here.

Ligneous conjunctivitis could present with pseudomembranous conjunctivitis, however it would be bilateral and not with the acute findings described in the vignette. **Vernal conjunctivitis** is due to seasonal allergies and would not be consistent with the acute presentation described. In addition, vernal conjunctivitis is typically bilateral.

Giant papillary conjunctivitis is another word for contact lens conjunctivitis. This would present as itching, an increase in mucous on the lens, and cobblestone appearance noted on eversion of the upper eyelid. A typical presentation is someone who slept overnight without taking his or her contact lenses out. So if you are wearing contact lenses and it's late at night and you are bored to the point you are *not* even producing tears, take out your contacts before falling asleep and waking up with giant papillary conjunctivitis

290) E) The absence of conjunctival injection or discharge rules out mucopurulent conjunctivitis. He is also afebrile and there are no other signs of periorbital or orbital cellulitis.

The description of erythema, edema and especially vesiculation is consistent with a diagnosis of contact dermatitis. The fact that it is not warm to touch or tender, while being pruritic further points away from an infectious etiology.

291) E) The most likely diagnosis of this patient is contact dermatitis and therefore the most appropriate treatment would be cold compresses and low potency mild topical steroid cream.

ANSWERS: ENT

292) A) With a low grade fever, a red eyelid that is warm to touch, and in the absence of chemosis, proptosis and blurred vision, the most likely diagnosis is periorbital cellulitis. Orbital cellulitis would require a much more toxic picture with more serious signs including proptosis and trouble with movement of the eyes.

There is no history of trauma making a corneal abrasion unlikely, plus the conjunctiva is none injected and no tearing is described. Without eye discharge and corneal injection, conjunctivitis is ruled out. The insect bite occurred 2 days ago making allergic reaction unlikely and simple periorbital cellulitis very likely.

293) A) For simple periorbital cellulitis the most appropriate treatment would be oral antibiotics to cover Staphylococcus and Streptococcus.

ENT

294) C) No effect at all. Expectorants have an effect by thinning out secretions under experimental conditions but not under clinical conditions. Since this is the clinical not the experimental boards, C is the answer.

295) C) All lymphoid tissue reaches maximum size between 5 to 7 years. This may be asked straight out or in the form of a graph where you will have to compare with the growth of other tissue.

It may help you to remember this coincides with them starting primary school, which comes in handy considering their exposure to all the other disease vectors, ahem children.

296) C) **A bark-like cough coupled with inspiratory stridor is typical of viral croup.** In addition, subglottic narrowing is the typical "steeple sign" seen on x-ray with viral croup. Epiglottitis is unlikely given the age of the child and their not describing fever or severe respiratory distress.

297) **E)** In a child of this age group, **unilateral foul-smelling nasal discharge** would be most consistent with a **foreign body.** There is no mention of the child being febrile, making sinusitis unlikely; besides, it would typically be bilateral, as would allergic rhinitis. Unilateral choanal atresia would present with non-purulent discharge. Juvenile angiofibroma would present with nose bleeding.

298) **A)** The combination of swelling over the postauricular area with outward and downward displacement of the pinna is virtually diagnostic for mastoiditis. Without any evidence of discharge, a *cholesteatoma* is unlikely, as are any of the other choices presented.

299) **B)** The *most likely* cause of a "sudden onset" of bilateral sensorineural deafness would be *viral labyrinthitis.* **In general, if something is of an acute onset and you had no idea of the answer, then a viral etiology would not be a bad choice.** The degree of severity and/or recovery is variable.

Autoimmune disorders are typically gradual in onset, and hearing loss due to drug toxicity would be gradual as well. The chances of a foreign body causing bilateral deafness would be unusual, especially when they are confirming that it is sensorineural.

300) **E)** Tympanometry measures tympanic membrane (TM) compliance and middle ear pressure. In most cases an immobile eardrum is caused by fluid in the middle ear. However, tympanometry in and of itself could not be used to diagnose otitis externa, otitis media, or the source of the middle ear effusion causing the decreased compliance. It also could not identify hearing loss, and certainly could not distinguish the type of hearing loss (conductive vs. sensorineural).

It only helps establish impaired mobility of the tympanic membrane which should be used with other clinical findings in establishing a diagnosis.

301) **C)** Penicillin remains the champion antibiotic to use for dental infections.

302) D) The most appropriate intervention in this setting would be to discontinue bottle feeding at night as well as nocturnal breast feeding. Both have been linked to development of dental caries in both age groups.

303) A) Hearing loss is the most common complication of otitis media. It is not clear if tympanostomy tubes help prevent hearing loss in chronic otitis.

304) D) The symptoms are consistent with a sinus infection. However the chronicity of symptoms makes for a diagnosis of chronic rather than acute sinusitis.

305) D) The red ear represents simple inflammation of the tympanic membrane. Pain management is all that is needed not antibiotics.

306) B) When conjunctivitis and acute otitis media present together, the likely pathogens are beta lactamase resistant organisms, making amoxicillin/clavulanic acid the most appropriate treatment of those listed.

307) C) The history is most consistent with gonorrhea pharyngitis and a throat culture for gonorrhea would be the most appropriate step in establishing a correct diagnosis.

Adolescent Medicine and Gynecology

308) D) Rapid refeeding of patients who are severely malnourished (which somebody who is 35% below ideal weight would be) can result in hypophosphatemia leading to potential cardiac failure, coma, and hemolytic anemia.

309) C) Factors associated with early initiation of early initiation of sexual activity include early onset of puberty, sexual abuse, and lower socioeconomic status. Factors associated with a later initiation of sexual activity include parental consistency, firmness in discipline at home and high academic achievement.

Access to condoms in school based clinics increased the use of condoms with intercourse but does not impact the rates of sexual activity or early initiation of sexual activity.

310) D) Adolescents have a limited ability to link cause and effect when it comes to high risk or unhealthy behavior including, seat belt use, overeating, smoking, and drug use. Often this behavior is a way of differentiating from their parent and obtaining a self identity. Therefore signing a contract with their parents will likely have an opposite effect. However adolescents do care a lot about their physical appearance and their physical performance. Therefore emphasizing the impact smoking will have on their athletic performance will likely had an impact in your attempts to get them to stop smoking.

311) D) Approximately 30% of gay youths have attempted suicide at least once; therefore depression and suicide ideation are not rare among homosexual teenagers. Transient homosexual experimentation is *not uncommon* in teenagers. Adolescents who are emotionally attracted to members of the same gender usually do *not* engage in sexual activity.

ANSWERS: Adolescent Medicine and Gynecology

312) D) Scoliosis inheritance is multifactorial not x-linked. It is more common in girls than boys and is defined as a curvature of the spine greater than 10 degrees. Adolescent idiopathic scoliosis is defined as scoliosis whose onset is seen in children older than 10.

Mild-moderate pulmonary compromise can be seen in spinal curvature greater than 60 degrees.

313) C) 25 % of sexually active adolescents become infected with sexually transmitted diseases each year. *Chlamydia trachomatis* and *Neisseria gonorrhea* can be asymptomatic in both males and females, and it is now possible to diagnose both through urine "amplification" techniques. These techniques are less invasive and should result in increased compliance and willingness to be tested.

314) A) *Hyper*thyroidism, *hypo*thyroidism, hyperprolactinemia and disordered eating can all result in anovulatory uterine bleeding. Cystic fibrosis would not be a significant consideration in the differential diagnosis.

315) C) The patient in the vignette is presenting with cyclical abnormal bleeding which is by definition, *menorrhagia*. Given the strong family history for the same, this is suggestive of a bleeding disorder. Of the 3 bleeding disorders listed, von Willebrand disease is the only one that makes sense. Factor VIII and IX are X-linked and primarily affect males.

There is nothing to suggest polycystic ovary syndrome or Crohn's disease.

Sports Medicine

316) D) Androstenedione, a testosterone precursor, is a schedule III controlled substance that is sometimes used as a sports enhancement medication. They bind poorly to androgen receptors and therefore, do not help with bulking up or any of the other effects users are seeking. So androstenedione is largely ineffective but still has the same negative effects as anabolic steroids.

These negative effects include **elevated** estradiol levels, **decreased** high-density lipoproteins (HDL), and **increased serum lipid levels. There is no increase in serum testosterone levels.** Therefore, they have the worst of both worlds: none of the benefits with all of the negative effects of anabolic steroids.

317)
1) B
2) C
3) A

Creatinine supplements are not recommended in kids under 18. The side effects include fatigue, abdominal pain, water retention, cramping and weight gain. You could be expected to be familiar with these side effects.

Anabolic steroid use results in muscle mass increase both through muscle hypertrophy and increased number of muscle fibers. Exogenous testosterone (Anabolic androgenic steroids are synthetic derivatives of testosterone) suppresses luteinizing hormone. Therefore, urine luteinizing hormone levels will be low resulting in an **increased** urine testosterone: luteinizing hormone ratio.

Guarana extract is used in energy drinks and is packed with caffeine. Therefore increased alertness, headaches and anxiety can result when using energy drinks containing large amounts of this extract.

ANSWERS: Substance Abuse

318) C) Maintaining an open dialogue and honest discussion often lowers the risk for a teenager using performance enhancing drugs. Encouraging appropriate nutrition and training is another method of deterrence by redirecting them to appropriate ways to improve performance.

Oddly enough, tests that reveal a low sperm count in teens who are already using anabolic androgenic steroids can be a motivator for teenage boys to stop using anabolic androgenic steroids. This would be the "kick in the nuts" method of deterrence.

Drug testing is not a proven method of deterrence.

Substance Abuse

319) C) Alcohol; had we asked, "What is the most widely used *illegal* drug?" the answer would have been marijuana.

Some might argue that love is the most widely used drug but it is not a registered trademark nor is it controlled by the DEA, as of this printing at least.

320) B) The physical findings are due to amphetamine which is adrenergic. This would explain the increased blood pressure, heart rate and the dilated pupils (**mydriasis**) and abdominal cramping.

There is nothing in the history to suggest undiagnosed bipolar disease. Alcohol and cannabis abuse would not present with this clinical history.

PCP abuse might present with tachycardia and hypertension but they would also need to describe hallucinations and/or slurred speech to distinguish from amphetamine abuse.

321) C) The patient is presenting with acute intoxication secondary to PCP and marijuana.

The clinical presentation of PCP intoxication depends on the degree of intoxication:

Low dose – mild inebriation

Moderate dose – catatonic blank stare, muscle rigidity, hypertension and tachycardia

Large doses – coma, seizure and respiratory distress

This patient is presenting with symptoms of moderate dose intoxication. The muscle rigidity can lead to rhabdomyolysis. If serum myoglobin is high enough there is a risk for deposition in the renal tubules causing renal toxicity.

Therefore the correct answer is to measure serum myoglobin.

Rectal Valium would not be a good idea in a patient who is catatonic with muscle rigidity for what should be obvious reasons. However IV Valium to relax the patient might not be a bad idea but was not one of the listed choices.

322) D) Drug use among high school students was at its highest in the 1970s this was followed by a decline in the 80's and then a gradual increase in the 1990s

Cigarette smoking among 8th-12th graders has *decreased* over the past decade.

The use of performance enhancing drugs *increases* the likelihood of use of other illicit drugs. Inhalant abuse is more prevalent among 8th graders than 12th graders

Among other risk factors for substance abuse alienation from conventional norms is one of them. Therefore homosexual adolescents have rates of substance abuse that are significantly higher than heterosexual peers.

323) D) High pitched voice, gynecomastia and pustular – papular acne would be a result of anabolic steroid abuse. The mood swings and mania would also be part of the presentation.

Growth hormone would not present with acne or the aggressive behavior depicted in this vignette.

ANSWERS: Disorders of Cognition, Language & Learning

Disorders of Cognition, Language & Learning

324) E) Most learning disabilities are life long and therefore continue into adulthood. Learning disabilities, which are very specific, do not reflect IQ and can therefore coexist with an above average IQ.

Learning disabilities are diagnosed based on history and neuro-psychometric testing.

Grade retention does not improve, and in fact may hinder, the progress of students with learning disabilities.

325) B) A child who can walk upstairs with one hand being held, can turn the pages of a textbook 3 pages at a time, can speak 10 words and can identify 1 body part is either an 18 month old child or a pediatrician who just completed 2 days of answering board questions and is headed home.

326) D) "Intellectual disability" (ID) is the currently preferred term for what was formerly referred to as "mental retardation".

Children younger than 6 years *suspected* of having ID would be more appropriately characterized as having *"global developmental delay"*

One exception would be in the context of a diagnosed recognizable syndrome associated with ID.

Close to **50%** of children with *severe* ID have **behavioral problems**.

Approximately **50%** of children with cerebral palsy will have some degree of ID.

Seizure disorders are approximately **10 times** more common in children who have ID.

The prevalence of sleep disorders is **inversely proportional** to **intelligence.**

327) C) Infants diagnosed with a syndrome known to be associated with intellectual disability become eligible at birth.

All other infants should be referred immediately when delays become evident. After age 3, toddlers should be referred to their local school system for services.

328) D) Dyslexia is a learning disability that results in difficulty with reading, spelling, writing, and with language in general. It cannot be prevented, but can be overcome with a variety of modifications. It is a disorder of language, not a visual deficit, therefore vision therapy is not effective. The best way to promote language development and reading skills is by reading aloud to a child with dyslexia. It has a multifactorial etiology, including genetic and environmental factors.

329) A) Activities that do not involve complicated rules and are non-verbal should be encouraged in children with autism spectrum disorder. Those that are individual and noncompetitive are definitely the best.. Lacrosse is a team sport involving complicated rules and extensive verbal communication with teammates. All the other listed activities would be much more appropriate and allow physical activity and enjoyment without stress for the child, the other players, and the families.

330) D) All newborns should be screened for hearing loss by 1 month of age and if they fail this screen they should have a comprehensive audiological evaluation by age 3. Early intervention services should be implemented by 9 months of age. There is no mode of communication that is more favorable, therefore auditory communication is not considered to be favorable to sign language. Early language developmental milestones such as cooing, pointing and social smiling can occur even in an infant with hearing loss. Therefore these signs are not reliable findings to rule out hearing loss.

331) B) This would be consistent with normal language development in a two year old child which is equal to (calculator please!) a 24 month old. This is easy to remember using the rule of 4s.

You should understand 1/4 of the language spoken by a 1 year old, 2/4 or one half the language of a 2 year old, 3/4 the language of a 4 year old and 4/4 or 100 % of the language spoken by a 4 year old. This alters during adolescence, until age 18 when you likely won't understand 1/2 to 3/4 of what they are talking about. This lasts a variable amount of time depending on your own ability to decipher that world.

332) C) Children who have difficulty saying or hearing the letter S, F or the th sound in English are demonstrating a difficulty with high frequency sounds which is suggestive of hearing deficit. Since this child was born outside the US it is not clear if he received a hearing screen as an infant as required in the US. There is no evidence of social anxiety or autism spectrum disorder. Coming from a bilingual household should not cause a specific finding such as this in two languages. This cannot be written off as normal language development.

Behavior and Mental Health

333) A) In this scenario, the depression is mild. Here we noted that the physical exam is unremarkable and the patient is otherwise healthy. On the boards, unless other contradictory information is presented, this is absolute. Therefore, in this case if we note that the physical exam is unremarkable and otherwise healthy, it is a fact.

The exceptions would be if there is information that is directly contradictory. In this case, they could be describing a finding that reveals the acute onset of a disorder. Another exception would be if something is in quotes, noted by a relative or someone who is with them. For example, if the grandmother notes that he has a "croupy cough". In this case you cannot, and probably should not, assume a diagnosis of croup.

Therefore, for this question, since he is otherwise healthy and the physical exam is unremarkable, lab tests would not be appropriate, ruling out choices B and C.

Mild depression that has not been treated with conservative measures such as psychotherapy or lifestyle change would not require psychiatric consultation nor would medications such as fluoxetine be indicated.

Therefore, the correct answer here would be lifestyle changes such as nutrition and exercise. This is also good advice if you are not necessarily depressed but feeling some fatigue and boredom reading through this book or in my case writing it.

334) A) Tics do occur with some variability with the start of some stimulant medications, but they are not a common cause of tics. This is due to stimulant medications lowering the threshold for developing tics. However, this association does not mean that stimulant medications are a cause of tics. Read the question carefully.

Nonstimulant medications such as atomoxetine are not always indicated when tics occur with stimulant medication. In fact, in some cases, the morbidity of the tics is a small price to pay for the improvement obtained with stimulant medication. Therefore, stimulant medication does not always have to be discontinued.

335) D) Dosing is based on clinical response rather than weight. Initial treatment with an extended release medication is often preferred over short acting. Baseline labs and EKG are not indicated routinely. However, periodic blood pressure measurements would be appropriate at follow up visit. Baseline labs and EKG would be indicated only when clinically indicated based on history or exam. If stimulant medication achieves targeted goals, then behavioral-modification therapy may not necessarily be indicated.

336) C) While some of the listed choices can be helpful such as individual psychodynamic therapy and school based interventions, the correct choice is **cognitive behavioral therapy**. This is a very practical approach that has a successful track record in treating mild forms of depression. This form of therapy includes techniques to reframe negative thinking, basically giving a new spin to negative thoughts. It includes goal setting and focusing on the future rather than rehashing past experiences typical of longer-term forms of therapy such as Freudian analysis, which is clearly the wrong choice for teenagers. Peer to peer file sharing therapy , well you can go ahead and fill in your own perverse innuendo.

337) A) You say **fluvoxamine**, I say **fluoxetine**. You can say what you want but if you want to be board certified, you better keep these psychiatric medications straight. Read the question carefully

Fluoxetine is approved for treating depression in children 8 and older.

Fluvoxamine and **sertraline** are not FDA approved for the treatment of depression in at any age. They are approved for treatment of obsessive compulsive disorder in children but for depression.

Escitalopram is an antidepressant approved for treatment of depression in children 12 and older.

Psychosocial

338) B) Emetine —the active ingredient in ipecac. Several keys in this question point toward Munchausen by proxy syndrome (MBPS). For one thing, she is ER-hopping in Central Connecticut despite the negative workup at what must be teaching hospitals in Manhattan.

A non-medical person using terms like "hypovolemia" and "capillary refill" is bizarre even for someone who has taken her kid in several times for a GI workup. One might argue that "maternal porcelain levels" would be the correct answer to diagnose a "crock". It is a tough one, but the questions do ask for the "best" answer to establish the diagnosis, not the most logical

339)
1) A
2) D
3) A
4) B
5) A

Night terrors occur during the first third of the night and the child is mobile during the episode, making for the possibility of physical danger. There is usually no recollection of the episode. There is often a family history.

With nightmares there is often vivid recollections of the scary dream. Neither one is associated with nocturnal enuresis.

340) E) While ADHD has no relation to diet, a well-balanced diet is appropriate advice for any child, regardless of diagnosis. There is no evidence that preservatives or any other food products including sugar causes ADHD.

341) E) This is a description of "disfluency" and is a normal finding in a child of this age and something the child will likely outgrow naturally with time. This typically occurs at the beginning of the sentence, especially when the child is tired or being asked a question. No further workup, studies, or intervention would be warranted at this time.

Ankyloglossia is the formal word for "tongue-tied". Even if this were present on physical exam, it wouldn't warrant any further intervention.

342) C) Intellectual Disability (formerly known as Mental Retardation) is a lifelong condition of significant impairment in condition and adaptive development. Normal IQ is 85-115 and the ranges drop by 15 points thereafter, so mild ID would be IQ 70-85, as in the patient in the vignette. This child would be expected to have good self-help skills as an adult, reach academic skills in the elementary school range, and achieve independent living and employability, but most will need some support and assistance.

Somebody with an IQ of 70 would be way overqualified to be an anchor on a political show on Sunday morning. Boredom would overwhelm them within a week.

343) D) The most common presentation for intellectual disability is language delay. The more profound the intellectual disability, the earlier this comes to the attention of parents, caregivers, and health care providers.[29]

---

[29] In many cases also known as physicians or PCPs (primary care providers).

ANSWERS: Psychosocial

344) **D)** Primitive reflexes are present at birth and through the first year of life, but are abnormal if they persist past that point. As the brain matures and an infant's development progresses, the primitive reflexes disappear as the infant gains fine voluntary motor skills. Persistence of primitive reflexes is seen in infants with cerebral palsy.

The *corneal reflex* is also known as the *blinking reflex*, where the eyes blink when touched or in the face of sudden bright lights. This reflext persists normally and is therefore not a primitive reflex.

In addition to the *step reflex* (touching the sole of the foot results in stepping motions; disappears at 1-2 months), other examples of primitive reflexes include:

Startle reflex – with drawing of the arms and legs in response to a loud noise

Moro response – elicited by partially lifting the upper body and letting go, resulting in the startled infant throwing its arms up

Parachute reflex – elicited by rotating the baby from supine to prone quickly, resulting in the infant putting its arms out

Tonic neck reflex – elicited with the infant laying supine and by turning the head to the side; the arm on that side extends out with the hand opened and the arm on the opposite side flexes with the fist clenched (Picture a *fencer* position and remember it well; this has been included in the photo section of the certification exam, and you need to know that it is a normal finding.)

Rooting reflex – when the infant's cheek is stroked it turns to that side

Grasp reflex – just as it says, the infant grasps an object placed in its hand and won't let go (disappears at 3 months)[30]

Primitive reflexes are *always* normal in males. In fact studies have shown that the number of primitive reflexes is directly proportional to testosterone levels.

345) **A)** Correction for prematurity should be done until the age of 2 years. In this case, if one adjusts for the 4 months prematurity and makes the assessment based on that of an **14-month-old**, then the mother need only be reassured since the milestones achieved would be normal for an adjusted age of 14 months.

---

[30] Normally reappears at law school graduation.

346) E) Head banging and thumb sucking in an 18 month would be a normal developmental variant seen in up to 20% of children between the ages of 6 months to 4 years, especially boys.

347) C) **Rolandic epilepsy** is characterized by seizures that occur at night. However, minor rolandic seizures are characterized by tonic clonic movements, often affecting one side of the face. A rolandic seizure typically begins at the corner of the mouth, and spreads to the rest of the face. Sometimes these seizures generalize to that entire side of the body. Clearly this is not occurring in the vignette.

Night terrors typically occur in boys between the ages of 5 and 11.[31] Night terrors typically occur during the first third of sleep during the *non-REM cycle.* Usually the child cannot be aroused and has no recollection of the event. Autonomic arousal manifested by tachycardia and tachypnea is typical.

348) D) There is often a lot of resistance on the part of parents to the diagnosis of ADD, and for good reason. There is a lot of misinformation out there and resistance for parents to accept and in some cases clinicians to make the diagnosis. On the other hand, the diagnosis is sometimes made flippantly, and stimulant medications are prescribed without employing the behavioral strategies needed to round out appropriate management.

Sometimes behavioral modification is employed without stimulant medication, often with poor results.

The **best approach** is to ease the parents into the diagnosis, reminding them that one can be successful.[32] A stepwise approach is best, with medication being discussed last, not first. Approximately 40% of children with ADHD will have an associated learning disorder, which may explain why the child in this case "doesn't like reading." This too must be addressed.

In fact AAP clinical guidelines require full neuropsychological testing to evaluate for other comorbidities.

---

[31] Thus it is always worth noting the gender of the patient.
[32] Adults with ADD tend to gravitate to fields like this father did because of the high level of stimulation and need for sustained attention.

ANSWERS: Psychosocial

349) **E)** Here, one would have to assume that the academic performance up until now has been fine, especially since they note that this deterioration was "recent". There is no evidence presented for focal brain abscess; hydronephrosis should not lead to uremia; and there is no evidence of a temporal lobe seizure or ADHD. Therefore, hearing loss secondary to recent aminoglycoside use would be the most logical choice.

Risk factors for aminoglycoside ototoxicity include: **therapy lasting more than seven days**, elevated serum levels, prior exposure to aminoglycosides, noise exposure, or high daily dose.

Therefore of the choices listed only hearing loss secondary to ototoxicity makes sense.

350) **B)** Sitting is usually achieved by 7 months, transferring objects by 6 months, and crawling and supporting weight and taking steps with assistance by 9 months.

351) **E)** This is a classic presentation of ADHD, a chronic condition that is frequently diagnosed around the first grade when greater demands are made. This child is exhibiting signs of hyperactivity[33] on physical exam. Difficulty completing homework assignments is an important feature of ADHD reflecting difficulty with organization skills.

Patients can often mask the signs during an initial evaluation. This is often not deliberate since the "novelty" of the situation is "stimulating enough" to keep the child focused during the evaluation.

Therefore, you cannot rule out ADHD in a child that sits still for the initial evaluation. In addition, on history the clinical signs must be present in at least two venues, typically at home and at school.

352) **B)** Clearly the mother is overextended and could use some assistance in handling her multiple responsibilities. Social work consultation would be most effective in developing strategies and tapping into resources that might reduce her stress level.

---

[33] Difficulty sitting still and talking excessively.

353) C) Children with special needs are at increased risk for physical abuse and neglect both at home and in educational and child care settings.

The divorce rate is *higher* than in families without a child with a special needs need.

Family members are at an increased risk for depression

Despite their experience, parents who are health professionals do not necessarily cope better than do parents who are not health professionals.

354) C) Crying for more than 3 hours a day more than 3 days a week for more than 3 weeks with no apparent reason is consistent with a diagnosis of infantile colic.

Colic begins as early as 2 weeks of age, usually peaks around 6 weeks of age, and tends to resolve around 4 months of age.

355) E) *Less than* 50% of parents enforce TV viewing limits for their children.

Around 50% of children 8 years and older have video game systems in their room and over 70% have TVs in their rooms.

The TV is on during meals in over 65% of homes.

The AAP does recommend that children younger than 2 years of age not watch *any* TV.

356) C) Studies have shown the strongest support for SSRIs such as fluoxetine when pharmacological treatment is necessary for the treatment of anxiety disorder in children.

ANSWERS: Critical Care

Critical Care

357) D) With the exception of hypoglycemia, all of the factors listed can interfere with an accurate pulse oximetry reading. Hypoglycemia can result in tachypnea but this should not impair oxygen saturation readings.

Carboxyhemoglobin absorbs the same amount of light as oxyhemoglobin therefore the combination is read as if it is oxygen and the reading is falsely elevated.

At high levels of methemoglobinemia, the pulse oximeter reads a saturation of 85%, regardless of the true percentage of oxyhemoglobin, therefore interfering with the accuracy.

358)
1) C
2) E
3) G
4) A
5) H
6) F
7) D
8) B

This is another board "grid" classic and bound to be on your exam. It should be an easy lay-up. It is best to take a systematic approach to this question. *Even though they say you can use each answer more than once this is rarely the case and you are best advised to cross out the answers as you select them.*

Respiratory acidosis, since you are dealing with acidosis, first look for a low pH, then a high CO_2.

Respiratory acidosis (compensated) will have similar CO_2 as uncompensated with a pH close to normal thanks to a rising bicarb.

Respiratory alkalosis will have a high pH and a low CO_2 along with insufficient compensatory low bicarb that has not impacted pH.

Respiratory alkalosis (compensated) will have similar CO_2 as above but with a low enough bicarb to bring the pH close to normal.

With the combined disorders you have contributions from CO_2 and bicarb pulling the pH **in the same direction**.

359) C) The fact that a child is stable in the ED is not the deciding factor regarding discharge and observation at home. Of the choices listed the only scenario where a child can be safely discharged home and observed is with a child submerged less than one minute not requiring CPR.

A child who required CPR, aspirated water, had a seizure, or had a change of mental status (such as a seizure), could deteriorate and needs to be observed in the hospital for at least 24 hours. Tachypnea could be a sign that acute respiratory distress syndrome and/or aspiration pneumonia could be developing.

360) D) In the past, *hyperventilation syndrome* was felt to be synonymous with *panic attack*. However hyperventilation can be triggered by other factors including change in position from laying down to standing. This would suggest increased baroreceptor sensitivity may be the cause in these situations not anxiety.

Hyperventilation syndrome is breathing in excess of metabolic requirements resulting in *hypo*capnia rather than *hypercapnia*.

It is very easy to see hypo and hyper as the same in the heat of the battle so pay particular attention to this when reading the questions *carefully*.

361) E) The clinical scenario is consistent with a diagnosis of meningococcemia. While ceftriaxone alone would be sufficient to treat this patient, you must also cover for the possibility of penicillin and cephalosporin resistant pneumococcus, Staph aureus, and enterococcus. Therefore the correct treatment would be IV Vancomycin *and* Ceftriaxone.

ANSWERS: Emergency Medicine

Emergency Medicine

362) D) Labial adhesions are rarely, if ever, related to sexual abuse; a crescentic hymen is a normal variation; and a normal genito-anal exam is frequently present in the face of sexual abuse and certainly does not rule out sexual abuse.

Physical exams for sexual abuse should focus on the labia minora and hymen. Tears that occur in the 3-9 o'clock/posterior position are more likely to be secondary to a sexual abuse.

363) D) Anteromedial tibia, 2 cm distal to the tibial tuberosity is the correct location. It is important to go 2 cm below the tuberosity to avoid the growth plate. The other choices are incorrect, especially mid sternum (ouch!).

A chicken bone might be one of the correct answers since this is where the intraosseous line is placed during PALS training.

364) 1) (E)
2) (D)
3) (B)
4) (A)

There are specific clinical presentations of abdominal pain which will be described which should make the diagnosis obvious on the exam.

Acute intermittent porphyria will be presented as paroxysmal abdominal pain along with headaches, dizziness, and syncope.

Ureteropelvic junction obstruction will be described as recurrent episodes of periumbilical and midepigastric crams with episodic vomiting.

Dysmenorrhea will be described as cramping midline abdominal pain.

Psychogenic pain due consistent with a conversion disorder will be described along with a psychiatric history in the patient and/or the family such as a labile patient and/or a depressed parent.

365) D) In most *hypertensive emergencies,* the drugs of choice are intravenous labetalol, nitroprusside, or sublingual nifedipine. **Patients with reactive airway disease are not able to tolerate a beta-blocking agents,** therefore beta-blockers are not the best treatment for hypertensive emergencies in asthmatic patients.

366) E) The first step in answering this question is to put the vital signs into descriptive adjectives. For example, this teenager is bradycardic and experiencing respiratory depression. This patient has the classic triad of opiate or narcotic ingestion **coma, pinpoint pupils, and respiratory depression**.

367) B) The technetium bone scan would be the most appropriate study to note any occult fractures missed by standard x-ray study.

368) B) Mannitol works via osmotic diuresis to reduce blood volume, and therefore works by reducing "brain water volume" overall.

369) D) Acute respiratory distress syndrome (ARDS) is a serious complication of "near drowning" in children. It is an uncommon complication, but is quite common on the boards.

The signs of ARDS may not be noted initially. During this "latent period", you may note mild respiratory distress, i.e., tachypnea, and perhaps an increased oxygen requirement. This is why "near drowning victims" who have required CPR in the field need to be admitted and observed even if they are clinically stable when they present to the ER.

On the initial physical exam you may note clear breath sounds or scattered rales. This is often followed by a typical deterioration as described in the vignette.

370) E) Anytime you are presented with the combination of bloody diarrhea and seizure you should think *"Shigella".* You can remember this by changing to "Shakella" to help remember that seizures can result in a child with *Shigella*.

ANSWERS: Emergency Medicine

371) **A)** With the exception of the child with purpuric lesions noted on the lower extremities, the other scenarios are consistent with non-accidental injury. Purpuric lesions on the lower extremity would be consistent with Schönlein-Henoch purpura, which is often mistaken for child abuse.

Any history of multiple fractures in the absence of an underlying condition such as osteogenic imperfecta would suggest abuse. The other injuries could not be explained as an accidental occurrence.

372) **C)** In any acute trauma scenario, follow the ABC rule, with "A" being Airway assessment and management. This is another case where reading the question is critical to see what they are asking. The key word here is "Initial". Had they asked, what is the "initial radiological" study to perform; it would have been computed tomography or C-spine series.

373) **C)** Bruises from accidental rather than intentional abuse can often be identified by location of the bruise for example the shins in toddlers. Minor injuries can indeed represent a pattern of abuse.

The age of bruise cannot always be determined by the color alone. Other factors including depth of injury, location and the skin color of the child also influence the color of the bruise.

Cultural healing practices such as "coining" have been well described and should be factored in when examining a child for possible abuse.

Burn marks in a splash pattern would be more typical of accidental injury rather than intentional immersion which would more typically present with a sock and glove pattern.

374) **A)** With a supracondylar fracture, there is a 1% chance of vascular compromise and a 7% to 10% chance of a radial or median nerve injury. However, these injuries do not involve the growth plate. They typically occur in a child who falls on an outstretched arm. They can present with pain in the forearm due to vascular compromise of the brachial artery, and attempts to extend the fingers results in pain.

These signs are more reliable than the presence or absence of a radial pulse. Therefore, *a supracondylar fracture is not ruled out with the presence of a radial pulse.* **Do not eliminate supracondylar fracture just because they note the presence of a radial pulse on physical exam.** Prompt orthopedic intervention is needed when this injury is suspected.

375) A) When injury to the abdomen is suspected (as is the case in the clinical scenario presented), an abdominal CT with contrast would be the most appropriate NEXT step. Serial hematocrits might be a good idea, but not the next step.

376) D) In any serious injury, the ABCs take priority. Therefore "assess airway" would be the most important initial step when assessing a fallen player with a potential cervical spine injury.

If the airway is compromised the facemask should be removed, while keeping the neck stabilized. **The helmet should never be removed in the field.**

In addition, you might want to note that the sport with the highest risk for cervical spine injury is football.

377) D) Rest, ice, compression, and elevation (RICE) are the most helpful 48 hours after the ankle injury. The most common cause of ankle injury is premature return not improper shoes or poor training. Fracture of the 5th metatarsal is commonly seen with inversion injuries. This should be obvious if you simply inverted your foot while answering the question.

Heat should not be applied initially after an injury. Cold packs, once again, should be applied for 48 hours following the injury as a part of (RICE)

378) C) Fentanyl has no anxiolytic properties and therefore must be used with an anxiolytic agent such as midazolam. Therefore it is used for procedures which are painful and would have a limited or no role in a procedure which is merely distressing and not physically painful.

Fentanyl has a shorter half-life than morphine and therefore, morphine would be more appropriate for a procedure that will be painful afterward.

Fentanyl definitely does play a role in conscious sedation in children. Why else would you be expected to know about it?

Fentanyl, if titrated too quickly or given in doses greater than 5 mcg/kg, can result in chest wall stiffness.

ANSWERS: Emergency Medicine

379) D) As tempting as it might be, reassuring comments such as "I'm sorry we have to do this" have been shown to increase not decrease anxiety in children about to undergo painful procedures.

Cartoons, breathing exercises, video games and music all are helpful distractors to reducing pain and anxiety during procedures.

If you chose A, B, C or E, "I am sorry to have to tell you that your chose the wrong answer", which is no more reassuring than getting a letter from the Board of Pediatrics that begins "We regret to inform you that … blah, blah … you may take the exam again next year."

380) A) 90% of allergic reactions to food in children are due to one of the following 6 allergens, milk, eggs, soy, fish, wheat and peanuts.

Serving a tofu, cheese, salmon, peanut omelette served on whole wheat bread would require inclusion of epi-pens with the table setting.

381) C) The most likely explanation for this clinical presentation would be Mallory Weiss tears. Bleeding due to a Mallory Weiss tear typically follows forceful vomiting.

382) A) Cyclic vomiting is by definition stereotypic recurrent episodes of nausea and vomiting with no identifiable organic cause. There are several features required to establish the diagnosis including 3 or more episodes of recurrent vomiting and intervals of normal health between episodes. There also must be a lack of lab or radiographic evidence to support an alternative diagnosis.

Amitriptyline and propranolol are effective *prophylactic* treatment. Antiemetic agents must be used during acute episodes.

Pharmacology and Pain Management

383) 1) (B) Acetazolamide.
2) (A) Furosemide.
3) (D) Hydrochlorothiazide.
4) (C) Spironolactone.

384) E) Trimethoprim/ sulfamethoxazole would be the first line treatment for each of the conditions listed except for exacerbation of chronic bronchitis for which it would be considered to be a 2nd or third line medication.

385) C) Valerian root is used to treat anxiety and insomnia. Caution should be used when taking sedatives or drinking alcohol.

386) C) St. John's Wort is used as an antidepressant and its mechanism of action is postulated to be serotonin reuptake inhibition, just like the SSRIs we all prescribe!

387) 1) (C)
2) (G)
3) (A)
4) (A)
5) (D)
6) (F)
7) (E)

Cyclophosphamide can result in hemorrhagic cystitis, therefore patient on this agent must be well hydrated. Patients on bleomycin need to be monitored for pulmonary fibrosis.

Both anthracycline and doxorubicin can be cardiotoxic. Vincristine is neurotoxic and asparaginase can cause pancreatitis. Methotrexate is associated with oral ulcerations.

ANSWERS: Research and Statistics

Research and Statistics

388) D) *Descriptive epidemiological studies* are performed based on case reports that suggest a pattern. They help establish a pattern, which can help define a hypothesis for further studies that would seek to determine causation.

Descriptive epidemiological studies do not "test" predefined hypotheses.

389) A) The sensitivity of a test is calculated by dividing the true positives divided by all of those with disease which is true positives plus false negatives

$$\frac{TP}{TP + FN}$$

The numerator is the total number of patients who test positive divided by the total number patients tested *with* the disease. The closer the result is to 1, the more sensitive the test is.

These tests are good for screening. Very few people with a given disease are missed. However, it can capture false positives. A good example of this is using ANA to screen patients with lupus. Very few cases are missed, but not everyone with a positive ANA has lupus

390) C) The specificity of a test is determined by the true negatives divided by the true negatives plus the false positives.

$$\frac{TN}{TN + FP}$$

The number of patients who truly don't have a disease are divided by the true negatives plus the false positives, which is the total tested population who do not have the disease.

Therefore, the closer this number is to 1, the more specific the test and the more reliable the result. A rapid strep screen is a good example where a positive result is reliable.

391) C) Case reports are just individual reports. They are the equivalent of reporting "suspicious" situations to the police but in and of themselves do not don't necessarily prove anything. However they do provide helpful " tips " the same way public reports provide tips for police detectives.

IF case reports present patients with rare findings with a common factor, it provides a clue regarding possible events causing the disease. It could identify correlation but will not prove causation. That requires more rigorous review and research to establish causation.

Anecdotal evidence and information reported by physicians would fall under this category as well.

This is probably how the idea that going out with wet hair causes pneumonia got started. Somebody a long time ago must have gone out with wet hair and "caught pneumonia". Then their neighbor noted that they also had a friend who went out with wet hair and "caught pneumonia" and next thing you know causation is assumed and generations of kids are told not to go out with wet hair.

392) B) Prospective cohort studies require a large number of subjects studied over a long period of time. This makes it a *poor* rather than an excellent method to study risk factors for rare diseases. The more rare the disease, the more subjects required to capture those who develop the condition being studied.

Given the large number of subjects that need to be studied over a long period of time, cohort studies are very expensive and time consuming. They are not good for studying diseases with long latency periods since this would mean following the subjects for an even longer period of time.

ANSWERS: Research and Statistics

393) A) The key to a correct answer here is memorizing the formula. In all likelihood, they will test you on either sensitivity OR specificity, but test on this concept they will. It is worth getting it straight so you can get one more question correct on the road to passing. The sensitivity of a test is the truly "positive results" over the total number with the disease, thus how "sensitive" a test is. Therefore it is:

[True positive test results] ÷ [Total with disease]

Just remember:

$$\frac{\text{True +}}{\text{Actual +}}$$

Total with disease would be all who have it, which are the *true positive* test results and the *false negatives*. In this case, the total number with the disease is 81 plus 37 = 118. The total positive test results are 81, and dividing this by 118 is roughly 0.68. Therefore, a very sensitive test (high number) will pick up a lot of patients with the disease and is therefore good for "screening". An example would be the rapid *Strep*, which is reliable when positive. Therefore, it makes good "sense" to use a sensitive test to "screen".

394) B) The specificity would be:

[True negative results] ÷ [Total without the disease (healthy)]

The total without the disease would be the true negatives plus the false positives (who are healthy). In this case, this would be 48 divided by (48 plus 5) 53 = 0.90.

This test is reliable to confirm the disease; for example *Strep* throat culture. Tests which have a high specificity, help **c**onfirm disease such as the throat **c**ulture for *Strep*.

395) E) This would be the positive predictive value, which is:

[True positives] divided by [Total positive test results]

In this case, it is 81 divided by (81 plus 5) 86 = 0.94. Positive predictive value is the chance of a person with a positive result actually has the disease.

As you might have guessed, the *negative predictive value,* which is not one of the choices here but could appear on the exam, would be:

[True negatives] divided by [Total negative results]

In this case, this would be 48 divided by (48 plus 37) = 0.56.

Now that you have waded through these questions, you should have an approach with high specificity and a high positive predictive value.

Ethics for Primary Care Physicians

396) C) The lime in the coconut therapy described[34] would come under the category of complementary alternative medicine or CAM for short. As their child's physician, you are under the obligation for beneficence, which is to act in the best interests of the patient. You are also under the duty for nonmaleficence which is to "do no harm". As long as this treatment is done along with traditional medicine, rather than instead of it, there is no reason for you not to explore this option with them. This would not betray your duties for nonmaleficence or beneficence. In doing so, you would be reviewing any side effects that might result from such treatment.

Choice B, you supporting what the *family* feels is in their best interests would be incorrect. First, treatment is based on what is in the best interests of the *child*, not the family. Ultimately, it is your role to determine *with* the family what is in their child's best interest. If you determined that their plan was not in their child's best interest you would not be obligated to go along.

---

[34] Yes that is the name of a song made popular in the early 1970s by Harry Nillson.

ANSWERS: Ethics for Primary Care Physicians

397) C) Palliative care is not exclusively for those with cancer nor is it exclusively geared toward helping families of children who are near the end of their lives.

Palliative care is primarily focused on helping families cope with life threatening conditions. Palliative care has been shown to improve mood and improve communication with health care professionals. Palliative care and life extending as well as curative treatments can, and often are, given together.

398) E) While drug testing the father may not be a bad idea and very tempting, it is not the correct answer. Drug testing a teenager at the insistence of the parents, with or without the patient's assent, would not be the first step. The first step would be to speak to the boy privately to see if drug use is an issue emphasizing that the discussion would be confidential.

Of course if the discussion revealed that the boy is at risk for harming himself or others, then confidentiality would not be applicable.

The main point is physician patient trust is key. Any correct answer should be a variation on talking to the patient in privacy and in confidence.

Any opinions regarding the Affordable Care Act should be reserved to discussion among peers who agree with you (and are therefore spot on in their opinion).

399) E) The American Academy of Pediatrics has deemed that pediatricians do have an ethical and professional responsibility to assist in the administration of justice in civil and court proceedings. However certain recommendations should be factored in. You are expected to testify in areas that are within your area of expertise. However, this is not the law, and the state cannot suspend your license for testifying outside your area of expertise.

Testimony should be based on current evidence based standards of practice related to the case, not necessarily your experience and practice in similar situations. One would hope these would be synonymous but regardless, your personal experience is not what should direct your testimony.

While one should spend the majority of one's time practicing medicine rather than testifying in court, this is not an absolute statement. For example, it would be appropriate for a retired physician to spend most of their time testifying in court.

One can receive compensation at a reasonable rate consistent with market value for the time spent on the case. It should never be contingent on the results of the case. Your opinion must be unbiased.

400) C) Accepting cash or any gift of large monetary value for personal use or gain is considered to be unethical. While it is tempting to accept such a gift, directly or indirectly through your friend Joey, it would interfere with any future doctor patient interactions you might have with this patient, or friends or relatives of this particular family. Making a donation to the hospital would not be of any personal gain.

Patient Safety and Quality Improvement

401) C) A near miss event is a potential adverse event which placed a patient at significant risk of injury but does not result in harm. It is important, since if it recurs in the future it could result in harm to the patient.

Near miss events can either be *intercepted* before impacting the patient or they can be *non-intercepted*. Basically these are "close calls" or "good catches".

By definition, non-intercepted near miss events do not result in harm to the patient. For example if a child received a dose of ibuprofen that was 3 times the indicated dose, it is unlikely that serious harm would result. Therefore choice C would be incorrect in stating that a non-intercepted near miss event **always** results in harm to the patient.

402) D) Adverse events occur in 1% of pediatric hospitalizations and 60% of these are preventable. Dosing errors are common and with increased technology there has been in increase in reported adverse drug reactions in the pediatric setting. The increase in reporting has been attributed to the increased ability to detect these errors and not necessarily to an increased incidence.

Traditional or folk remedies can certainly have harmful interactions with standard medications. This is especially the case on the boards, so pay close attention when you are given a question that involves a home remedy that is chipped off a tree. You might as well replace the word home or folk remedy with skull and crossbones poison.

The risk for adverse drug events is **3 times higher in *pediatric* hospitalization** when compared to adult hospitalizations. This should make sense since adult medications are "one size fits all" and in our world dosing is always weight dependent, making for a much higher risk for error.

ANSWERS: Patient Safety and Quality Improvement

403) D) Premature administration of vaccines and over immunization is a common errors when immunizations are administered by multiple clinicians, especially in multiple settings. The risk for poor coordination is higher. Template based e-prescribing decreases the risk for medical error. Templates often incorporate patient weight, documented drug allergies and concentrations. These reduce the risk for human error. In addition, electronic notes also reduce the risk for handwriting error in the rare case where a doctor suffers from mild dysgraphia. That is of course rare!?

Medical errors in the ambulatory setting are definitely not limited to medication and immunization errors. Mislabeling of specimen and ordering incorrect labs are also very common medical errors. Home measuring devices are far inferior to well-marked syringes for reducing dosing errors at home.

Unfortunately, lower level of parental education increases the risk for not understanding medication instructions and administering medication incorrectly to a child.

404) B) Limitations on resident hours has definitely reduced fatigue. Having trained during the "golden age" of the 36 hour straight shift I can only hope so! However, these limitations have also resulted in an increased number of sign offs, each one increasing the risk for error in communication. Of course fatigue can increase other errors, including decreased doctor safety when driving home on no sleep but that is not what the question asked!

The root cause of 60-70% of sentinel errors are due to communication errors. Performing sign out at the bedside with patient and parental involvement decreases risk for error. It also decreases parental perception of risk. Standardization of sign off predictably decreases communication errors.

405) B) This would represent a "near miss intercepted event". Near miss *intercepted* events are errors that are intercepted before reaching the patient. In this case it was likely due to a keyboard stroke error by entering methadone instead of methylphenidate. In this case the pharmacist "intercepted" the error converting it into a near miss.

A near miss non-intercepted event would one that was not intercepted but no harm or injury was caused to the patient. An adverse drug event or ADE would be an error that results in an injury to the patient. There was no harm or injury to this patient since you were given the opportunity to correct the error. In this case it was a good thing you were neurotic enough to go back to your office to make sure the door was locked. Now you can go play your round of golf and go hiking with Phil.

References

Growth and Development

1. Jaffe AC. Failure to thrive: current clinical concepts. *Pediatr Rev.* 2011;32(3):100-107.

2. Cooke DW, Divall SA, Radovick S. Normal and aberrant growth. In: Melmed S, Polonsky KS, Larsen PR, Kronenberg HM, eds. *Williams Textbook of Endocrinology.* 12th ed. Philadelphia, PA: Saunders Elsevier; 2011:935-1053.

3. Marks KP, LaRosa AC. Understanding developmental-behavioral screening measures. *Pediatr Rev.* 2012;33:448-458. DOI.

4. American Diabetes Association. Standards of medical care in diabetes—2013. *Diabetes Care.* 2013;36 (Suppl 1):S11-S66.

Poisoning and Toxins

5. http://www.who.int/selection_medicines/committees/subcommittee/2/charcoal_rev.pdf

Research and Statistics

6. Godless F. Applying research evidence to individual patients. BMJ. 1998;316:1621–1622.

Patient Safety and Quality Improvements

7. Woods D, Thomas E, Holl J, Altman S, Brennan T. Adverse events and preventable adverse events in children. *Pediatrics.* 2005;115:155–160.

8. Neuspiel DR, Stubbs EH Patient safety in ambulatory care. Pediatr Clin North Am. 2012;59(6):1341–1354.

9. Cox ED, Carayon P, Hansen KW: Parent perceptions of children's hospital safety climate. BMJ Qual Saf. 2013;22(8):664–671.

10. Morrell RC. JCAHO revises standards to help reduce medical errors. *APSF Newsletter.* 2011;16(2).

Ethics for Primary Care Physicians

11. Ref: Is there a role for palliative care in progressive pediatric neuromuscular diseases? The answer is "Yes! J Palliat Care. 2008;24(4):265-269.

12. American Academy of Pediatrics, Section on Hospice and Palliative Medicine and Committee on Hospital Care. Pediatric palliative care and hospice care commitments, guidelines, and recommendations. Pediatrics. 2013;132:96.

13. Ref PIR January 2015.

14. American Academy of Pediatrics Committee on Medical Liability. Guidelines for expert witness testimony in medical malpractice litigation. Pediatrics. 2002;109:974.

15. American Academy of Pediatrics Committee on Medical Liability and Risk Management. Expert witness participation in civil and criminal proceedings. Pediatrics. 2009;124:428.

Notes

Notes

Notes